EVE'S RIB

EVE'S RIB

The Groundbreaking Guide to Women's Health

MARIANNE J. LEGATO, M.D.

THREE RIVERS PRESS

NEW YORK

Published by Three Rivers Press, New York, New York.
Member of the Crown Publishing Group, a division of Random House, Inc.
www.randomhouse.com

THREE RIVERS PRESS and the Tugboat design are registered trademarks of
Random House, Inc.

Originally published by Harmony Books, a division of Random House, Inc., in 2002.

Printed in the United States of America

Design by Lauren Dong

Library of Congress Cataloging-in-Publication Data
Legato, Marianne
    Eve's rib : the groundbreaking guide to women's health/ Marianne Legato.
        1. Women—Diseases.   2. Women's health services.   I. Title.
RC48.6 .L44 2002
616'.0082—dc21   2002024120

ISBN 1-4000-4829-X

10 9 8 7 6 5 4 3 2 1

First Paperback Edition

For Christiana and Justin

Acknowledgments

Writing this book was tremendously enhanced by the following people:

Harmony Books' Shaye Areheart, who convinced me that the lay public needed and would welcome the new information about gender-based medicine, and who believed I could write *Eve's Rib*.

Richard and Leslie Curtis, whose encouragement, multiple readings, and intelligent critiques helped me polish, focus, and sculpt the final manuscript.

Peter Guzzardi, my line editor, who cajoled, pummeled, and urged me on until the last line in the last paragraph of the last chapter made coherent sense.

Christiana Killian, whose readings—and rereadings—of each chapter prompted some of the best suggestions for clarifying my thoughts I could have had.

John Pepper, Myron Weisfeldt, Craig Wynett, and T. George Harris—the four men who made the Partnership for Women's Health at Columbia University a reality.

Christine Haider and Palesta Fitzgerald, whose loyalty, support, and skill are vital to the research and educational mission of the partnership.

My patients, who have taught me so much.

Contents

Introduction

Eve's Rib is not just about women's health, but about the health of both sexes and the new science of gender-specific medicine. Until now, we've acted as though men and women were essentially identical except for the differences in their reproductive function. In fact, information we've been gathering over the past ten years tells us that this is anything but true, and that everywhere we look, the two sexes are startlingly and unexpectedly different not only in their normal function but in the ways they experience illness.

As a rigorously trained biomedical scientist, I've always been interested in the excitement of exploring a new idea and finding out how to prove it true or false. Until the last decade, we've made the assumption in medicine that it's necessary to study only men, and that the data we harvest can be extrapolated to women without modification. To a certain extent, the assumption was forced upon us: studying women, particularly premenopausal women, is not without risk both to the subject herself and to a fetus that might be conceived during the course of an investigation. Thus, we've found it difficult to recruit women for study unless their reproductive years were behind them, and those supporting research have been justifiably wary of incurring huge damages as a consequence of harming an unborn child. Furthermore, because of the cyclic variations in younger women's hormonal levels, any investigation that included them would require larger numbers of them than of men to really come to a firm conclusion about whether or not gender differences exist. So we've excused ourselves—and women—from including them in biomedical investigation on the grounds of its being too dangerous and too expensive—even unfeasible in terms of finding sufficient numbers—to do so. But all that has begun to—and must—change.

It has been women themselves who have demanded a change in the way American scientists and doctors do business. With an increasingly more coherent and powerful voice, women have forced the federal government and the biomedical establishment it supports to define the differences between males and females. The results have been nothing short of astonishing. As we compare men and women, we are finding that in every system of the body, from the very hairs of our heads to the way our hearts beat, there are significant and unique sex-based differences in human physiology. The new data are transforming the way we prevent and treat disease. We are refashioning our male models of health and illness by asking questions we never even would have framed until we studied both sexes. The answers to those questions are turning out to be completely unexpected and fascinating.

We haven't solved every problem about the difficulties in studying women, particularly those still involved in building their families. But as the Belmont conference observed, it is a principle of justice that if women are to share in the benefits of medical research, they must also share in the risk that research inevitably entails when we are testing the safety and usefulness of a new drug or intervention. Every woman who wants more attention to her health must be willing to help harvest the new information and bear a personal responsibility for helping to generate credible answers to the questions that we are asking.

Somehow, Eve's gift of an apple to Adam became a metaphor for our banishment from an ideal world of perfect harmony to an existence troubled with suffering, sorrow, and eventually death. The reality is quite the opposite. If we are courageous, persistent, and intelligent about using Eve's gift to expand the new science of gender-specific medicine, the next decade of research will inevitably produce significant improvements in our ability to improve and lengthen human life. *Eve's Rib* explains why.

Eve's Rib

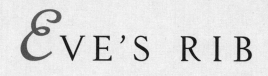

CHAPTER I

Eve's Question: "How Am I Different from Adam?"

U NLESS THEY ARE focusing on the reproductive system, most doctors have a tendency to treat patients as though they were all the same sex: male. We consider patients' stories of their illnesses, examine their bodies, and interpret their laboratory tests as though gender were irrelevant. We even write prescriptions the same way, seldom considering patients' size or body composition, let alone sex, to determine how their bodies will process and use a particular drug. Even our understanding of what makes men and women different has been simplistic. (Many doctors ascribe it all to hormones, which is only partly correct.) In short, we've practiced medicine as though only a woman's breasts, uterus, and ovaries made her unique— and as though her heart, brain, and every other part of her body were identical to those of a man. It's not that the profession is overrun with poorly educated sexist practitioners. For the most part, rather, it's the way we have been educated, as though women were simply small men and data we have about the male body were the standard for both sexes. Most of the information doctors use in diagnosing and treating disease was gathered almost entirely from research on males. Remarkably, it's only recently that medical science has begun to grapple with the complex factors that define a person as male or female.

The notion that women and men are essentially interchangeable isn't new. If you want to know what a culture holds to be most important and true, read its myths. Consider the story of Adam and Eve. As the crowning glory of the newly created world, God transforms some clay into the first human—a male, perfect in every way. In spite of the abundant richness of Paradise, however, Adam is lonely. Consider God, on the fifth day, taking pity on Adam. He puts him into a deep sleep, takes some tissue from his side, and fashions it into a woman. It's not only a biblical tale, it's also a medical fable, and an eerily prophetic one at that; it describes the first anesthesia, major surgery, and cloning of a new individual. More important, it tells us that Eve is literally derived from the stuff of Adam. Apart from their reproductive biology (which is admittedly unique for each, a fact with which the story's author never grapples), by definition Adam and Eve are identical: Eve is simply a smaller version of Adam.

Still, she is different enough, apparently, to want to explore beyond the boundaries set for them both: she wants more information; she wants answers to questions that only she has formulated. She tempts her hapless mate into an ill-fated collaboration to acquire that knowledge (which, she is assured by Satan, will give her more power over the world around her)—and they are expelled from Paradise, condemned to a life full of effort, pain, and all the other assorted ills of the human condition. Although we can't know precisely what she wanted to ask, I've always imagined that one of her questions was this: "How am I different from Adam?"

Eve may have brought about our exile from Eden, but perhaps she set the precedent for a minor medical revolution as well. The fact is, women have never really accepted the way doctors do business. All too commonly, when a woman would report to her doctor that a medicine made her palpitations worse instead of calming them, or that the pain from her heart attack had centered in her stomach rather than in her chest, he might simply tell her, "I've never heard of that" (or in an academic medical center, the more formal "We don't see that"). He might add to himself, *Your reactions are obviously the result of some emotional issue. I can't take your complaints—or you—seriously.* But thankfully, women have continued to ask their questions, and more and more they are insisting on answers.

I met some of those women personally for the first time in 1992, when I left my laboratory to go on a nationwide book tour publicizing *The Female Heart: The Truth About Women and Coronary Artery Disease,* which I wrote with Carol Colman, a medical journalist.[1] In ten days I spoke with hundreds of women about their experiences with coronary artery disease and the important ways these experiences differed from those of male patients. They told me a shocking number of stories about doctors' dismissing them as hysterical or "anxious" when they were asking for help with what turned out to be their first heart attack. Every time I gave a talk, I was met with a barrage of challenging questions for which I had no answers. Those ten days with these women, who were so hungry for information about their particular needs and their unique experiences, changed my life. At the end of that trip, I returned to my fully funded laboratory, locked the door, and gave the key to the scientist next door.

My own research on coronary artery disease had shown that males and females experience that disease very differently; now I wondered, might the experience of other illnesses besides coronary artery disease differ between men and women? For that matter, what about differences in normal function? What if the biological sex of a person affected all the baseline measurements and standards that are accepted as "normal" for a healthy human? If it did, doctors would have to modify the way they've always thought about medicine. Our society might even have to construct entirely new strategies for preventing and curing disease, strategies that would emerge from a new awareness of the fundamental differences between men and women.

SEX OR GENDER: WHAT ARE WE TALKING ABOUT?

What is it, precisely, that makes people either men or women? It's more than just hormones; it's a whole variety of things, and scientists are only just beginning to tease out the various ingredients of what biological sex is, and why males and females are different. But the complex interplay of genes and hormones that define biological maleness and femaleness is only half of the story. Males and females don't exist in a vacuum, and the way they develop and thrive—or fail to thrive—

is a very real consequence of the societies and cultures in which they find themselves. Biological sex is overlaid by the roles, rules, and expectations society sets for its members. The combination of our biological sex with the impact of our environment on our health and behavior as men or women is called gender. Health is affected as much by environment as by genes and hormones, and it can be virtually impossible to determine whether biology or the way people live in their particular communities is responsible for their health. If Muslim women get malaria less often than Muslim men, is this because their immune system has some innate, sex-determined ability to fight off infection, or because they are required to wear clothing that conceals them from head to toe—and thus protects them from the bite of the mosquito carrying the malarial parasite? If African women get trachoma (a parasitic infection of the eyes that destroys vision) more frequently than African men, might it be because women spend much of their day at the river's edge, where the parasite lives, doing the family laundry and socializing with other women of the community? Teasing out these differences is one of the most complex and difficult challenges modern science faces.

WHY HAVE RESEARCHERS STUDIED ONLY MEN?

Like every other scientist trained in a top-rank medical center, I was taught, and had accepted, that the results of research done in males were applicable to both sexes. In anatomy laboratory, none of my instructors thought it important to point out whether our cadaver was male or female, except when we studied the reproductive organs. I didn't even entertain the idea that there might be significant differences between the two beyond the reproductive system. In a revealing monograph,[2] the National Academy of Sciences' Institute of Medicine calculated that fully two-thirds of all diseases that affect both men and women have been studied exclusively in men. As a result, the models not only of how humans function normally but also of how they experience illness are essentially male. This assumption that men and women are so alike that it's not important to study women directly has dominated the way scientists do biomedical research and the way doctors practice medicine. Until very recently, everything about American health care, from research protocols to public health policies, reflected an intellectual mistake of astounding proportions, one that undoubtedly has affected the health and the lives of many women over the years.

How in the world did this happen? The answer is complicated. It is not simply that men, who have traditionally dominated the worlds of academic medicine and scientific research, didn't care about women or thought they were unimportant. In fact, many of the dictates that restricted medical research to males were the result of an effort to protect women—particularly premenopausal women, whose reproductive abilities were of primary concern—from the risks of experimentation. (Scientists seldom if ever worried about a young man's reproductive potential: society still measures men principally by what they achieve, and women by their ability to conceive and bear children.) Researchers know that damage done to a fetus conceived during a clinical trial is not only an ethical issue; it can have potentially disastrous legal and economic implications if the child is born malformed.

This philosophy of protectionism, by the way, was reinforced by the publicizing of Nazi atrocities during the Nuremberg trials, particularly the Doctors' Trial, which detailed the experiments done on concentration camp inmates (including children) in the name of medical science. That exploitation was not exclusively the work of fringe elements in the medical profession. One of the doctors, Paul Rostock, was the dean of the University of Berlin School of Medicine and chief of its department of surgery. Before the war, he had been an internationally respected member of the scientific research community, but now it was clear that even the "best" doctors were capable of exploiting the defenseless and the vulnerable in the name of medical progress.

The Nazis were not unique: events in the United States reinforced the need for protection of vulnerable populations. In 1963 a physician-researcher injected cancer cells into elderly patients at the Jewish Chronic Disease Hospital in New York, in some cases without the consent of the physicians responsible for their care, and in other cases over the objections of doctors who pointed out that the patients were incapable of understanding what was going to happen to them.[3] In 1932 in the Tuskegee Syphilis Study, doctors withheld treatment for syphilis for years in four hundred black men, so that doctors could observe the natural course of the untreated illness, even though it was known that penicillin cured the disease. This famous example of the abuse of unprotected research subjects took place well before the Nuremberg trials.

Concern for pregnant women (or young women who might become pregnant during the course of a drug trial) as subjects of medical research was fueled by two disasters. In the 1940s and 1950s, diethyl-stilbestrol (DES) was a popular drug used in pregnant women to prevent miscarriage (in spite of excellent evidence from well-done studies that it really had no ability to do so). In the 1970s it became apparent that many daughters born of those mothers were suffering from a rare form of vaginal cancer. A second drug, thalidomide, an antinausea treatment approved for use in 1958, produced devastating deformities in children born to women who used it while they were pregnant. These tragedies were a major reason that Congress in 1962 passed protectionist legislation (the Kefauver-Harris amendments and the National Research Act), which created a commission to develop guidelines for research in human subjects.[4] Careful principles were developed and encoded in the policies and procedures of the National Institutes of Health.[5]

Another reason that only males were used in clinical studies was scarcity of research dollars. The cyclic variations in women's hormonal levels made it necessary to include many more of them in any protocol in order to achieve significant and reliable information. Researchers viewed men as a more homogeneous and stable population and were reluctant to spend extra time and money to study females.

Today all of this is changing. Scientists know that in most cases the benefits of including women in clinical trials and research studies far outweigh the drawbacks; they know more about how to include women in studies without putting them at risk; and they are beginning to understand the importance of the information. They have arrived at this position via a couple of routes: tragedies like the thalidomide disaster; the increased influence and effectiveness of the feminist movement; and revolutionary improvements in medical technology. A societal event also greatly influenced the change.

HOW WORLD WAR II CHANGED AMERICAN MEDICINE

Exploring the factors that have shaped modern medical science and women's place in it could be a life's work, but the historical event that is widely accepted as playing a pivotal role in the process is World War II. The workforce changed during the war, and women took on all kinds of jobs that were once the exclusive province of men. These changes took place not only in factories and offices but in the medical profession as well. For the first time in history, women were admitted to surgical and orthopedic training programs and rose to high positions in teaching hospitals. When the war ended, they were often sent back to specialties like obstetrics and pediatrics, where "women belonged," but they never returned to prewar roles and attitudes.

The war also profoundly increased the power of physicians. Before the war, physicians, armed with little more than laudanum, whiskey, and leeches, were unable to do more in the face of disease than cultivate the clinical skills that made the best of them superb diagnosticians, with a precise knowledge of how a disease, once contracted, played out its natural course. Their primary function was to predict a patient's fate: "On the tenth day of this pneumonia, the patient will either die, or her fever will break and she will recover." But under the pressures of the battlefield, physicians refined and used the first antibiotics to combat infection. They perfected the new discipline of plastic surgery (begun by John Converse, private practitioner and faculty member of NYU College of Medicine, on the battlefields of France during World War I) and discovered that a virus was the cause of the hepatitis that they inadvertently spread when transfusing wounded soldiers with contaminated blood. They learned how to treat shock and to safely anesthetize patients during long surgical procedures.

By the end of the war, Americans had developed an almost religious respect for the power of science. In 1944 scientists in the U.S. Public

Health Service led Congress to pass the Public Health Service Act, which greatly expanded federal funding for medical research. Between 1955 and 1968, under the direction of James A. Shannon, the National Institutes of Health expanded significantly. By the 1960s, the United States led the world in medical and technological advances.

By the 1980s, pushed by a growing and ever more effective voice from American women, the U.S. government was paying a great deal of attention to women's health. In 1985 the Public Health Service issued a report on women's health issues, concluding that the "historical lack of research focus on women's health concerns has compromised the quality of health information available to women as well as the health care they receive."[6] This profoundly important acknowledgment spurred the NIH to announce a year later that no research on a disease that affected both sexes would be federally funded unless it included female subjects.

Unfortunately, a 1990 General Accounting Office report indicated that the NIH was not implementing its own policy. A survey of fifty current grant applications found that 20 percent of them gave no information about the sex of the research population; over a third proposed to include women but did not specify precisely how many of the study subjects would be female; and several proposed to look only at men, without any justification for a single-sex design.[7] As a result, the NIH founded the Office of Research on Women's Health, which Congress gave legislative authority and permanent status by the National Institutes of Health Revitalization Act of 1993. By that year the Food and Drug Administration had reversed its 1977 protectionist policy excluding premenopausal women from drug trials and had established new guidelines about how to include them safely.

In short, the world of scientific research has undergone a sea change in its attitude about research in women. A new principle, very well expressed in the NIH's 1979 *Belmont Report*,[8] emphasizes the concept of *justice* in selecting research subjects. According to this principle, one subgroup of the population (men, for example) should not have to bear the risk for everyone else in a clinical trial; if women might benefit from a new drug or intervention, they must share the possible dangers involved in testing its safety. I often point this out to women enraged that "doctors have only studied men! When will scientists begin to learn about our problems?" Women who want the benefits of carefully supervised and planned investigations into their unique physiology must agree to bear the dangers, risks, and responsibilities of participating in those investigations.

Like the rest of society, women have reaped the benefits of medicine's increasing expertise. They now not only reach menopause but also survive and live beyond it. A baby girl born today is expected to survive until eighty-six; by 2015, 45 percent of American women will be forty-five or older. They will live a full third of their lives after the cessation of their reproductive potential. Their compelling problems will involve not childbearing but the latter-day plagues of cardiovascular disease, osteoporosis, and dementia. These women, born in the postwar period, are setting the tone for the present health care discussions in the United States.

ANSWERING EVE'S QUESTION:
BUILDING A NEW RESEARCH PROGRAM

Even after the success of my first book, about the differences in how men and women experience coronary artery disease, I knew that leaving the research career for which I had been trained so carefully and for so many years would be a risky business. I remember sitting in a tiny diner on a Sunday morning seven years ago and telling my mother I was going to close my laboratory, where I had built a successful career studying how the heart develops from uterine to adult, independent life. She was horrified. "You'll have to prove to me—and to Columbia's Department of Medicine—that there are enough differences between men and women to make this new research worthwhile. And who is going to fund you to do that?" She had something there. The only currency in an academic medical center, especially one as sophisticated and preeminent as Columbia, is facts: not only did I have to convince my chairman that I was on to something, but I had to find the money to support what I wanted to do.

In fact, I succeeded in building a program to learn more about women because of the help of four men. The first was my chairman, Myron Weisfeldt, a charismatic scholar who had been the president of the American Heart Association and who knew me well. (Waiting for my appointment with Dr. Weisfeldt, I remember feeling as Columbus might have felt while waiting for his first audience with Ferdinand and Isabella, hoping to convince them of the economic bonanza that would result if his notion that the world was round turned out to be true.) I told him I believed I could help convince the academic community that research on women was not only possible, but mandatory: it would prove to be fundamentally important to achieving better health for both sexes. In spite of overwhelming general skepticism about the idea, and doubts among my colleagues about the economic feasibility of such studies, Weisfeldt agreed to help me. Within days I had a small office and an even smaller salary. But I was freed from all my heavy teaching obligations, and my only assignment was to find major funding for what I was proposing: a program devoted to studying the differences between men's and women's normal function and in how they experience disease.

In a second stroke of good luck, T. George Harris, founder of *Psychology Today* and one of the judges who had given my first book the Blakeslee Award of the American Heart Association just months before, called to ask me if I would be interested in becoming a consultant in women's health to Procter and Gamble. P&G had just entered the pharmaceutical business and wanted to understand the impact of the burgeoning interest in women's health on its new venture. I met Craig Wynett, head of Corporate New Development for P&G, with whom I felt an immediate and exciting kinship. I knew that this was my opportunity to find real funding. If I was correct, I explained to Craig, companies like his stood to benefit tremendously from the new science, with the opportunity to develop a whole new generation of gender-specific products. It was a thrilling idea for both of us.

Within weeks, I was invited to lunch with John Pepper, then chairman and CEO of P&G. A quiet, courtly man, he wasted no words. Even as the soup was served, he asked, "Do you have the confidence of your university?" (Read: "Are you some wild-eyed romantic here on your own because a few of my staff think you might have an interesting idea, or are you speaking for Columbia as a properly credentialed faculty member, supported by one of the greatest and most respected American universities?")

Grateful to be swallowing soup and not something more substantive, I considered that the "confidence of my university" was restricted at that moment to my chairman, who was playing long odds in betting that what I was proposing would actually turn out to be real and important. By the end of lunch, I had made enough inroads to meet my next real test: a proposal to the scientists of P&G, a group of more than fifteen hundred Ph.D.'s and M.D.'s, that gender-specific medicine was a worthy idea with a real future, and that product development, from toiletries to medicines, would be substantially benefited by a better understanding of the differences between men and women. My most vivid memory of that first meeting with Pepper was what he said as dessert was served. "I want to pick up *The Wall Street Journal* in ten years and read that Procter and Gamble has done more to advance women's health than any other company in the world. This is not just about moving more boxes of our products across the counter." Not only would this particular company pay more attention to women for the right reasons, but Pepper would make a personal effort to expand support for this new program beyond his own company, even to competitors. After giving Columbia $2.5 million to begin the research, Pepper and Wynett personally brought me to the executive offices of Dow, Nike, Bristol-Myers Squibb, Pfizer, and Johnson & Johnson to form a consortium of support for our idea, which we named the *Partnership for Women's Health at Columbia University.* We're now in our fifth year, and studying the differences between the sexes has proved fruitful beyond my wildest dreams.

LEARNING ALL ABOUT EVE

Doing this research is a little like being in California during the gold rush: it's hard to resist working at top speed. Everywhere we look, we find a new wealth of information, and we are confirming far beyond our expectations what women seem to have known all along: they are not small copies of men. Women have a unique biology, with unsuspected but far-reaching differences. Our research makes it abundantly clear that sex is a vitally important determinant not only of how humans function normally but also of how they experience disease. And it is prompting new questions that might never have been asked had we not used gender as a basic variable. Here are some examples:

• Diabetic women are less likely to suffer from osteoporosis than nondiabetic women. This unexpected finding has sent us back to the drawing board to find out more about diabetes and its impact on bone biology. On the other hand, diabetes puts women at tremendously increased risk for coronary artery disease (CAD), *even if they are relatively young and still menstruating.* For reasons we don't understand, while diabetic men have a doubled risk for CAD, a diabetic woman's risk is four to six times *higher* than that of normal women. Why does diabetes apparently catapult women's cardiovascular system into old age? If we could answer that question, we would have a much better idea of why and how CAD develops in the first place and develop better ways to treat it in both males and females.

• Hormones have profound effects on the way men and women metabolize drugs. For example, epileptic women often have seizures just before or on the first day of their menstrual period. Similarly, asthmatic women often have attacks at the beginning of their menses. Doctors who understand this will be able to adjust the dosage for a woman who complains that her epilepsy or her asthma is worse right before her period—and not chalk it up to her imagination.

• Men and women have important differences in their immune systems. A prominent pharmaceutical company developed a vaccine against the herpes virus, then discovered that the vaccine was effective in women but not in men. Because this finding had important economic consequences, it was reported in *The Wall Street Journal.* The next time a company invests in developing a vaccine, it will take some time to examine how it actually operates in the people who are going to use it. (Sometimes my patients come in during the winter with influenza in spite of the fact that I've given them a flu shot. I'm now keeping track of their sex—a new clinical experiment, albeit on a tiny scale, that I never would even have thought of doing had I not read the *Journal*'s account. You might tell your own doctor about this: if you get sick despite having had a flu shot, the cause may be not a bad batch of vaccine, but your gender-specific response—or lack of it—to the inoculum.)

• On the whole, men and women have small but real innate differences in their brains. For example, men produce 52 percent more of a hormone needed to prevent depression (serotonin) than women. This hormone is an important link between our experience and our emotional state, a fact that has tremendous implications for treating depression: social success, like a job promotion, increases serotonin concentrations in the brain. Success literally does go to your head! The fact that women are, on the whole, twice as likely as men to be depressed may account for their relatively less important place in many societies. Instead of prescribing an antidepressant, a doctor might suggest counseling, focusing on the issues in a woman's life that are demanding more effort than feels comfortable or appropriate. It may sound too simple to be true, but a new job that ensures better use of your talents and gives you more independence and control over your day might actually increase the levels of serotonin in your brain and relieve your depression.

• When their serotonin levels drop, women tend to withdraw and become anxious and reclusive. Men, on the other hand, respond to low serotonin levels with aggressive behavior and often increase their alcohol intake. Your symptoms of depression might be very different from your husband's: while he may increase his drinking or become uncharacteristically short-tempered and abusive, you may find it difficult to leave the house, or have panic attacks in a crowded department store. Ask your doctor to help you decide if your real problem is depression. Similarly, a husband or son whose drinking is spiraling out of control may need more than a reprimand or a referral to Alcoholics Anonymous. (Note: No doctor should ever dismiss the symptoms of a patient as evidence of an inherent weakness or inadequacy.)

• Childbirth profoundly affects a woman, changing her metabolism and leaving her susceptible to postpartum depression. But it affects men as well, producing biological changes in new fathers. If you're pregnant, just before your baby is born, your husband's level of cortisol (the stress hormone) will surge, but it will drop rapidly just after the birth (hopefully leaving him calmer and more serene!). At the same time, his testosterone levels will decrease and his estrogen levels will rise—perhaps, the evolutionary biologists tell us, making him more interested in the newcomer and more comfortable with staying near home to protect and support you and the baby.

• Doctors sometimes make different decisions for men and women with the same illnesses. Across the board, women are less likely to receive aggressive medical treatment for heart disease than men and are less likely to receive kidney transplants for end-stage renal disease. They are less frequently diagnosed with chronic obstructive pulmonary disease, a chronic disease of the lungs that is usually caused by smoking. (Yet cigarette smoking is as common or more common among women than in men, and women lose lung function more rapidly with smoking than men.) Hundreds of women have told me unbelievable stories about how they were patronized and dismissed by doctors, both male and female, who simply didn't respect their symptoms as genuine. Recently, as I concluded a luncheon talk about heart disease in women, a member of the audience rose to say that she had been having chest pain whenever she ran or climbed stairs. She was a doctor's wife, and her husband sent her to his colleague, a cardiologist. After hearing her story, the cardiologist told her that women didn't get heart disease at her age (she was forty-two) and said, "I'm going to call your husband and tell him to take you away for the weekend and give you what you really need. You'll be fine after that." With tears of rage in her eyes, the woman concluded her story: "A month later I had my first heart attack."

This is an enormously exciting time in medicine. Doctors are beginning to take care of patients with an entirely new appreciation of their physiologies. As in all research, however, our most effective teachers are our patients. Above all else in my work, I love the consulting room, where the sick person explains to me how it feels to have her disease. The patient lays on my desk the clues about what's bothering her, like pieces of a puzzle that we must both put together into a coherent whole. I am never absolutely certain we've gotten the right answer. Together we test my idea of what's wrong, correcting and expanding the story until we agree on a working hypothesis and decide on a reasonable course of treatment. The quickest way to arrive at a wrong conclusion, I've found, is to dismiss the patient's story as bizarre or ridiculous. Because doctors have been trained in a tradition that has studied only men's stories of illness, we must take exceptional care with our observations of illness in women, as observation is one of the primary ways we will be able to learn. As colleagues of mine have said in amazement: "Everywhere you look, there's a difference!"

Eve's apple was anything but the poisoned fruit for which Adam had to pay a terrible price. Using gender as an important variable in medical investigation is producing completely unanticipated new data and is raising new questions, and the answers to those questions will be valuable to everyone. Studying women as we study men isn't solely a matter of political justice, let alone of pandering to feminist angst. It is an intellectual imperative and will produce better, longer lives for both sexes. With a little luck, scientists will have the backing of businesses interested in this "new science" and its unique marketing opportunities. Companies are increasingly intrigued by opportunities to make more effective, gender-specific products for men and women, such as toothpaste for the special needs of menstruating or pregnant women, or a drug that will stabilize, without hazard of death, an arrhythmia to which women are particularly susceptible. In short, we are at the beginning of a new era: the era of *gender-specific medicine.*

While this science is still very new, I want to share with you what I have learned from my research and the research of my colleagues. This book will take you, chapter by chapter, through the new information about sex-specific differences in all the major systems of the body. It will help you understand that the differences in men's and women's biology extend well beyond reproductive function. My hope is that you will reap two rewards. First, you will have more confidence in your own experiences and will be more comfortable telling your doctor what you are feeling, even, if need be, challenging attempts to minimize or deny your symptoms. Second, you will learn vital information about how men and women differ—information your doctor may not know. For example:

- Women are more likely than men to recover their speech after a stroke.
- Women are susceptible to potentially lethal arrhythmias when they take some of the very medications that *stabilize* cardiac rhythm in men.
- The symptoms of a heart attack for a woman may appear more like indigestion than a cardiac aberration; misdiagnosing this problem can cost her her life.
- Asthma, arthritis, epilepsy, migraine, diabetes, and depression all can worsen just before menstruation, but a simple adjustment in medication can prevent most of it.
- It is more dangerous for women to smoke than for men. For the same number of cigarettes smoked, women are 20 to 72 percent more likely than men to develop lung cancer.
- Women feel pain more intensely than men, particularly pain from pressure or an electrical shock. Women are also more likely to have pain at a distant site from the part of the body with the problem. (This is called *referred* pain.)
- Sexual dysfunction in men *and* women may respond to testosterone.
- Osteoporosis isn't a disease of older women alone; back pain in an older man will prompt a savvy doctor to order a bone density test, just as he would for a woman.

It's not simply that information like this may improve the quality of your life and the lives of those you love. Knowledge, as Eve suspected, is power. The more widespread this information, the more doctors will be prompted to keep learning about gender-specific medicine, to train medical students differently, and to urge pharmaceutical companies to use gender as an important variable when they design new products.

Medicine in this century will be practiced with an entirely new understanding of the differences between men and women. I expect that within the next five years, the first gender-specific medical practices will be opened: not "women's health centers," devoted exclusively to treating only one sex, but places devoted to the meticulous comparison of data about both sexes. For example, instead of looking at breast cancer in isolation, we will consider men with breast cancer a national resource and invite them to participate in gender-specific research so that we can explore the sex-based differences in this illness and better understand how to prevent, treat, and cure it. Our patients are our real teachers, the best opportunity we doctors have of improving the quality of care for everyone.

CHAPTER 2

The Brain

⁓

WHEN I WAS five, I asked my surgeon father—whom I considered the font of all knowledge—what my IQ was. After a brief silence, he answered me with a single trenchant sentence: "Intelligence is the ability to manipulate the environment." I found that answer then, as now, fascinating. How we assess the world around us, and how we use experience to meet its challenges successfully, is one of the most interesting questions in all human biology. How do we become who we are? How do we remember things, file away experiences, learn new skills, grow in expertise?

Neurologists today are providing us with fascinating and provocative insights, one of which merited the Nobel Prize in medicine for 2000: *experiences actually change the anatomy of the brain.* From instant to instant, the physical shape of our nerve cells (neurons), the chemicals that we use to send messages from one neuron to another (neurotransmitters), and even the very molecules that make up the brain are all in flux. Each of our experiences is transmitted to our brain cells, stimulating the formation of new proteins, which actually increase and strengthen the connections between neurons. With repeated stimulation, whole networks of neurons develop that are specialized to process that particular kind of information. This translation of experience into structural changes is referred to as brain *plasticity.* It is how we learn; how we experience and interpret our environments; how we develop a history and an identity. It is how we become *experienced,* learning to fear some places, people, and circumstances and to delight in others. No matter how mystical and ephemeral our thoughts, feelings, insights, and emotions may seem, they are all consequences of physical events produced by our neurons and the communications between them.

How does all of this happen? And does it happen differently in men's brains than in women's? Are there essential differences in the brain that depend on biological sex?

SEX AND BRAIN STRUCTURE

Until recently, neurologists have assumed that the brain's anatomy is identical in men and women, as with just about every other organ of the body. But the more we look (especially if we believe that there might, in fact, be something to find), the more we discover real differences in human organs as a function of biological sex. The brain is no exception.

The shape and size of the brain, as well as the numbers of its cells and the extent to which they are interconnected, differ between men and women. Scientists call these differences in anatomy *sexual dimorphism* (*di* means "two" and *morph* means "shape").

Both animals and humans show sexual dimorphism in brain size and shape. Men's brains are generally 15 to 20 percent larger than women's, but women's brains contain about 11 percent more neurons in one very specialized area of the cerebral cortex, just behind the eye, that is involved in recognizing tonal differences in language and music. Women also have more extensive connections between neurons and between the two halves of the brain than men. The right hemisphere of the brain, which houses the ability to understand the properties of three-dimensional objects in space, is larger in men. The left hemisphere controls speech. Other parts of the brain have differences that are mirror images, from hemisphere to hemisphere, depending on gender: the inferior parietal lobe (the part of the brain directly above the ear) is larger on the left in men and larger on the right in women. This part of the brain processes the information we receive through vision and touch. In the hypothalamus (the part of the brain that helps control hormonal levels), there is a collection of cells called the sexually dimorphic nucleus, which has almost twice as many cells in males as in females.

It's well and good that neuroscientists have catalogued these differences and that they have, in some instances, a general notion of how they affect behavior, but what do they really understand about the genesis of these differences and why they should exist at all? The process is akin to assembling a jigsaw puzzle in the dark—scientists have identified some of the pieces and have even pushed a few together, but they haven't really gotten a look at the whole picture.

Some sexually characteristic differences are determined before birth, as we know because differences in the patterns of interneuronal connections aren't changed by postnatal hormonal influences. In animals, such differences can be caused before birth only by castrating males or by giving testosterone to females early in fetal development. Other differences in the size of some parts of the brain do occur under the influence of hormones in postpubertal life. Parts of the hypothalamus, for example, are larger in heterosexual males than in transsexual and homosexual males. These differences are not present at birth; they appear at only about four years of age and disappear again after fifty or sixty. Scientists believe these changes are the result of a complex interaction between experiences and hormones, a phenomenon we're only just beginning to understand.

While we know that men's and women's brains have dramatic and very significant structural differences, we don't know whether those differences translate into differences in behavior, aptitude, or cognition. Most of our information about brain sex differences comes from research in animals, where it is evident that not only the *structure* or shape of different parts of the brain but also certain *behaviors* are sex-specific. For example, the mating behavior of some species differs dramatically: the brilliantly colored South American male cowbird struts his bright plumage and sings loudly to attract the female, whose own tunes, if she sings at all, are neither as loud nor as complex. In the males who have the most complicated and loudest songs, a part of the brain called the vocal center is much larger than in the female.

But people are not songbirds, and the question of whether differences in human brain structure make men and women *behave* differently or have different talents is much less clearly answered. Certainly anatomical differences could explain some observed behavioral differences between the sexes; for example, if men's brains are larger as a result of their inability to prune back extra (or defective) neurons during development, perhaps retaining damaged cells makes them more susceptible to impaired brain function in response to brain damage early on. On the other hand, the fact that men have more neurons may explain the earlier onset of dementia in women—the latter simply have fewer brain cells and are more impacted by their loss than are men. But at the moment, these ideas are only speculations—and exciting new hypotheses to test.

PROBING THE LIVING BRAIN

Thanks to powerful new techniques, neuroscientists are making enormous progress in mapping the anatomical *and* functional differences in the brains of men and women. Most of the information about the brain that I learned in medical school came from anatomists, who looked only at brain structure, and from physician-scientists, who matched—usually at autopsy—the damaged area with the patient's specific defect.

The classic and groundbreaking case in brain mapping is that of Phineas Gage, a laborer in the late nineteenth century whose brain was pierced by an iron stake in a dynamiting accident. Incredibly, he survived, but he was "never really the same"; in fact, even after his wound had healed completely, his wife and co-workers found him almost intolerable. Gone was the quiet, hardworking day laborer; in his place was a rowdy, moody brawler prone to fits of rage. Gage's wound was probably in the frontal lobe, in the part of the brain responsible for regulating emotion and affect. Another classic brain-mapping example is a patient whom Paul Broca studied; the patient couldn't speak and was found upon autopsy to have damage in a small area in the front of the left side of the brain. Broca assumed, correctly it turns out, that this area was involved in the production of speech; to this day, we call this brain part "Broca's area." Carl Wernicke, using an associative technique, showed that another part of the brain is involved in picking the right words for communication. Wernicke had a patient who could speak but whose sequence of words (some of which were even made up) made no sense.

Neuroscientists owe a great debt to these early pioneers in the field, though the information from their crude if ingenious methods provided only a tiny part of the story. Today powerful new tools can simultaneously investigate both the structure and the function of the intact, living brain in real time, while patients are performing various activities and following commands. One of the most exciting is a noninvasive procedure called *functional magnetic resonance imaging* (functional MRI). Functional MRI can identify the areas of the brain that are associated with, for example, producing intelligible speech or developing an emotional response to a stimulus. One of the most important ideas that the new techniques have yielded is that no one specific location in the brain controls complex tasks like speech; rather, several areas may be involved. Even more intriguing, *depending on the sex of the subject, those areas may be quite different.*

Among the most accomplished investigators using functional MRI to sort out unique features of male and female brains are Sally and Bennett Shaywitz at Yale University. Their pioneering work has shown for the first time that quite literally *men and women use different parts of their brains while thinking.* They asked subjects to decide whether various nonsense syllables rhymed; the men's brain activity was restricted to a small part of the left hemisphere near Broca's area, while women used another area in addition located in the right side of their brains. Confirming this finding, Sandra Witelson at McMaster University in Hamilton, Ontario, has shown that this particular area of the right brain is larger in women than in men. Using the same technique as the Shaywitzes, Ruben Gur at the University of Pennsylvania School of Medicine found that even at rest men's and women's brains function differently: men's limbic system (part of the brain involved in the experience of emotions) had higher activity in the portions thought to be involved with the perception of motion and action, while women's limbic system was activated in newer, more recently evolved areas that have to do with the interpretation of expression and the nuances of speech.

Why do these differences exist and what implications might they hold for our understanding of male and female behavior? We do not know, but we have made astonishing progress in our understanding of the gender-specific brain and how it develops.

HOW DOES THE BRAIN BECOME MALE OR FEMALE?

At the beginning of its development, the fetus is neither male nor female, but early in the first trimester the sexes begin to develop differently. By the sixteenth week of life, in females, a tubular system called the Müllerian duct develops into a female genital system, complete with ovaries. In males, the Y chromosome activates the manufacture of a hormone that promotes the development of testes. Both the ovaries (when the fetus is three months old) and the testes (when the fetus is two months old) begin sex-specific hormone production.* It is these sex hormones that make the brain either male or female by acting on its developing tissue at what is called a *critical period*, a brief period of time in development during which the brain is responsive to hormonal influences.

Hormones do not influence the brain as straightforwardly as you might think. Testosterone does not masculinize the fetal brain directly but enters the brain cells, where an enzyme† called *aromatase* converts it into estrogen. Paradoxically, it is actually high intracellular concentrations of estrogen, formed from testosterone, that make the brain male. Without testosterone, there is not enough estrogen to impact the developing tissue. Maternal estrogen cannot act on the growing fetal brain, even though a great deal of it circulates in the fetal bloodstream;

---

* Testosterone is not exclusive to males; women's ovaries make small amounts of it. Similarly, estrogen is not the exclusively "female" hormone; the testes also produce it. It is the relative amounts of these hormones that are sex-specific; females produce more estrogen and males more testosterone. But both sexes have both hormones throughout life.

† An enzyme is a chemical that changes the speed of a chemical reaction without itself being changed in the process.

somehow the fetus is protected from its mother's estrogen. Even the fetus's own estrogen does not seem to penetrate the fetal cell very effectively. Without high intracellular levels of estrogen, then, the brain develops into that of a female.

Some scientists believe that the female brain is "neutral," a default outcome that results from a developmental pattern that is not affected by hormones at all. Others believe that estrogen actively influences the development of the female brain but that much lower concentrations are required than those for the male brain to produce its sex-specific structure and function. In any case, through this marriage of genetics and hormone production, the brain is "hardwired" to be either male or female long before birth.

Continuing Brain Differentiation After Birth

Sex-specific development continues through puberty and is maintained by hormonal action for the rest of our lives. The differences in our brains remain apparent until old age, when they become less striking. It isn't an exaggeration to say that the brain is as sexual an organ (if not more truly so) than the ovaries or testes.

At birth and during the first years of life, as the brain grows it undergoes periodic bursts of new cell formation, but as growth continues, many of these cells are "pruned back" and disappear. Interestingly, the developmental bursts occur in different parts of the brain at different times, probably critical times when input from the outside world can have an important and lasting impact on the brain function. If kittens are deprived of sight for the first three months of life by sewing their eyelids shut, they never regain vision, and parts of their brain development are stunted. This doesn't happen to adult cats, whose brains are no longer in that window of time in which sensory input has such a dramatic developmental impact. Such periods of opportunity probably happen throughout normal postnatal life. Special skills or talents may suddenly appear: mathematicians, for example, develop their peak ability quite early in their lives. An enriched environment probably enhances the abilities of the developing infant, but scientists don't know how, what, and when to present to the child to maximize its potential. Certainly infants living in deprived environments suffer from behavioral and intellectual handicaps, but for the most part the development of an infant is a reasonably sturdy process, relatively resistant to either the poverty or the richness of the environment.

Boys have larger brains than girls at birth, but boys are much more susceptible than girls to developmental disorders of the brain like mental retardation, impaired understanding of language, stuttering, autism, Tourette's syndrome, tic disorders, attention-deficit/hyperactivity disorder, and nighttime bedwetting. Emese Nagy and associates at the University of Texas in Houston use something they call the "gender paradox" to explain this phenomenon: although boys have larger brains than girls, they point out that newborn boys also have lower metabolic rates—their body temperatures and heart rates are lower than those of newborn girls. This means that their brains may have a greater need for oxygen and energy and, simultaneously, a relative inability to provide it. Nagy believes that this paradox may explain the greater occurrence of all these disorders in males.[1]

DO MEN AND WOMEN HAVE DIFFERENT INTELLECTUAL ABILITIES?

What about differences in intellectual ability and talents between men and women? Are they attributable to gender differences in brain structure? Unfortunately, this issue is so emotionally charged that many experts simply refuse to discuss it; others do so only very cautiously. Current science does indicate, however, that while no significant difference exists in overall intelligence, there are tiny but real differences between men and women in particular intellectual abilities and talents. Whether these differences are learned or are "hardwired" into the structure of the brain is very difficult to say. Most of the data about sex-specific thinking patterns and abilities come from animals, but there are striking parallels between what we find in rats and monkeys and what we observe in humans. The scientists who have just finished the definitive monograph from the National Academy of Sciences' Institute of Medicine[2] on gender-specific science point out several things about observed differences in the abilities of men and women:

• There's a *marked degree of overlap* in specific abilities between the sexes; the most dramatic differences occur at the extremes, with the most talented individuals, rather than over the bulk of the population. For example, most world-class artists are men, although there are exceptions; among the Impressionists, Mary Cassatt certainly held her own. The same is true of celebrated composers and conductors, who are principally male.

• When mean scores for a particular task are calculated, the differences between men and women are significant, but they are smaller than the differences between the highest and lowest scores for people of the same sex.

• Observed differences between the sexes *may apply only to a certain stage of life and disappear over time.*

• *How a particular ability is measured* can affect the result depending on the sex of the subject. A recent study showed that women are less able than men to solve spatial problems, like working through a maze, if the testing is done with virtual reality systems, as in the training of astronauts. But additional factors that we have not yet discovered may be modulating these abilities.

Even with these qualifications, though, some real differences exist in the *overall* intellectual ability of men and women. These include the following:

• Women have *superior "verbal abilities,"* including spelling, grammar, fluidity of speech, writing, vocabulary, and oral comprehension. Women are not better at all components of verbal ability, but in any of these areas, where there is a superior performance, it is women who best men.

• Women *remember things* better than men, whether verbal or nonverbal. For example, they are generally better at memorizing telephone numbers and at using landmarks to find their way back to a specific location.

• Women perform *finely coordinated movements* better than men; they can even repeat tongue twisters more fluently and accurately than their male counterparts.

• Boys' ability to outperform girls in *mathematics* is striking. In Scholastic Aptitude Test (SAT) math scores above 500, boys do better than girls two to one; over 600, five to one; and at 700 or above, a whopping seventeen to one! Critics of these measurements point out that mathematical skills depend significantly on experience, and that more boys than girls are enrolled in advanced math classes. When the data are corrected for this one variable, the differences are actually much smaller, although boys still beat girls. In general, the two sexes seem to approach math problems with different strategies and abilities. Boys excel when they use spatial relationships, shortcuts, or choose among several alternative paths to solutions, whereas girls excel when the answers depend on verbal skills or remembering and understanding classroom-based information. It may be, then, that the alleged superiority of men in mathematics may have to do with the fact that they have more flexibility in strategic decision making than do women.

• There are differences in the way men and women remember the events of their own lives: women are more likely than men to recall childhood memories, particularly if they are associated with emotion, either in themselves or in others.

• Women are more sensitive than men to facial expressions.

• Men are better able to understand the movement of three-dimensional objects in space. For example, when men and women are asked what happens to the level of water in a glass when it is tilted, most men have the correct answer (the surface of the water remains parallel to the ground because of gravity), but one in two women get it wrong. Male and female rats learn tasks that have to do with spatial relationships quite differently. Just as with humans, female rats use landmarks to help them learn a new path, while males do not, even when they are available. (When her neighbor asked my daughter how to find the home of a mutual friend, she answered, "Go down Madison Avenue until you hit Prada, then turn left.") Even more interesting, when men and women were asked to negotiate a maze in a virtual reality laboratory, functional MRI imaging techniques showed that men used the right (the "spatial" side) while women used the left (the "language" side) of their brains to complete the task.[3]

• Some scientists report that women's ability to solve spatial tasks varies with the phases of their menstrual cycle. During menstruation, when estrogen levels are lowest, women have the most success with such challenges. Others have found that women with congenitally high levels of testosterone have an improved ability to perform spatial tasks. In contrast, when men experience a drop in testosterone, they lose some of their ability to solve these kinds of problems.

WHAT BEHAVIOR IS LEARNED AND WHAT'S INNATE?

Many women don't want to hear that their brains are different from those of men. It has taken centuries for us even to begin to catch up with the opportunities men enjoy. My daughter could be a brain surgeon if she chose to, but when I went to medical school thirty years ago, I never even considered the idea; brain surgery was for the men in my class.

Are the differences between men and women "hardwired" into our brains, or do they exist because of the roles society assigns to us? How much about us is inevitable and how much is learned? Do girls become "motherly" because they're given dolls to play with? Are they less physically active than boys because they're taught to be "ladylike"? My daughter recently observed a striking exchange between a mother and her four-year-old son on a New York street corner. The little boy's eyes were brimming with tears, and he was clearly upset about something. "Boys don't cry," his mother chided him. "You might as well begin to understand that right now. So just suck it up." As adults, when men don't talk about their emotions, is it because they have learned not to or because an impassive response to something troubling is hardwired into their brain? A colleague of mine, New York pediatrician George

Lazarus, believes that in spite of our best efforts to train them, girls and boys are different from the outset. He tells a story of parents who were determined to give their daughter the same opportunities as their sons and not to "close off" potential vocations by gender-specific lessons. They bought her four trucks to play with, and she received them enthusiastically, but one day neither she nor the trucks were anywhere to be found. Finally, her mother discovered her in her bedroom. As her mother entered, the little girl signaled her to be quiet. The trucks were placed carefully in a row on the pillows of the girl's bed, with the covers drawn up over them. "Shhhh, Mommy! They're sleeping," she explained.

Every society sees boys and girls differently from the moment they're born. They are valued differently and treated differently, and they are expected to play different roles and, in many instances, to achieve quite different goals. Our biology and our experiences combined define what we are, and we all have learned lessons that profoundly shape our behavior. The simple fact of being male or female is layered over with lessons about how males or females are valued and expected to behave in society. Separating what's due to sex from what's due to gender identity is often impossible, which makes it difficult for researchers to be certain about how immutably different men and women actually are. But as investigative techniques improve, scientists are becoming more certain about which differences are functions of biological sex and which may actually be a result of the ways a culture treats men and women.

Is Our Sense of Gender "Hardwired" into Our Brains?

The fact that the brain is at least anatomically male or female early in development has provoked a tremendous amount of speculation about whether a person's sense of sexual identity and of sexual preference are immutable, and whether doctors are justified in "reassigning" sex in individuals born with ambiguous genitalia. William Reiner, a urologist at the Johns Hopkins Children's Center in Baltimore, has described a group of 27 children who were born with normal male chromosomes

(X and Y) and normal testicles (indicating normal exposure to testosterone in the uterus) but no penises. All but two were castrated at birth and raised as girls, but in spite of this attempt to "reassign gender," they all acted like boys in their rough-and-tumble play patterns. Fourteen of the 25 castrated children reassigned their own gender and said they were actually boys, one as early as five years old. The two children who were reared as boys were less psychologically maladjusted than the others and were well accepted by their male peers. This study would indicate that the "genderization" of the brain in the uterus produces a person's sense of self as a man or woman, even when an environment "tells" the person precisely the opposite. Even being castrated at birth and raised as the other sex cannot change this inner experience of maleness or femaleness; it is "hardwired" into the brain.

More support for this notion comes from other variations in development. A defect called *congenital adrenal hyperplasia*, for example, causes girls to have an excess of male hormones. These children have a block in the chain of events through which the adrenal gland makes its final product, cortisol. The chemicals that are made early in this chain of events resemble testosterone and are masculinizing. If their hormonal balance isn't corrected, these girls may be so masculinized that their enlarged clitorises may be mistaken at birth for penises. At puberty, their ovaries begin to produce estrogen and they develop breasts and begin to menstruate. Nevertheless, exposure of their brains to these abnormal adrenal hormones during development has masculinized these girls. Indeed, although they apparently think of themselves as female, they engage in a great deal of activity thought to be more usual for boys and are characterized as having "tomboyish" behavior. As adults, several of them are not only uninterested in having children but actively dislike the idea of caring for children.

Another developmental anomaly also lends credence to the "hardwired" theory. There are genetic males (with an XY chromosome pair) who produce normal amounts of testosterone but whose bodies have no receptor for the hormone. (A receptor is a protein that functions as a "lock" into which a "key," in this case a hormone, fits.) An individual may produce plenty of testosterone, but without a receptor he/she can't use it. The person matures as a female, because the normal testis also produces small amounts of estrogen. At puberty, in fact, breasts develop, and the person becomes sexually active as a female, but lacking a uterus never menstruates. Since the brain was never masculinized *in utero,* the person not only looks like a female but *feels* like one, even with an XY chromosomal pair. This indicates that in spite of male or female genetic equipment, *hormones* and their prenatal impact on the developing brain provide the critical factor that makes us feel—and behave—like men or women.

Transgendered people are individuals who have no unusual features in their complement of hormones, in their hormones' relative concentrations, or in their genitalia, yet feel that they are essentially the other sex. Conceivably, the usual timing or biology of their intrauterine brain development was somehow changed by a problem like maternal malnutrition, maternal stress, or maternal ingestion of some drug. Some scientists have suggested that homosexuality might be the result of a variation in the process of intrauterine brain genderization. Existing data certainly suggest that that might be the case, at least for some individuals.

In fact, maleness and femaleness may not be as immutable as was once thought. While we assume that sex is a result of whether a person has an XY or an XX chromosome, the hormones that are the consequence of that genetic equipment clearly have a profound and irreversible impact on gender identity. This impact is well substantiated by the natural experiments in children who develop without hormonal receptors for testosterone or have had intrauterine exposure to the excessive amounts of testosterone that I've just described. Maleness or femaleness is extremely fluid in other species; several kinds of fish *change sex in response to their social rank!* For example, when a male blue-headed wrasse (a coral reef fish) dies, the largest female in the group immediately begins to act like a male fish, actually converting to a male (with fully male gonads) within days. Other kinds of fish are hermaphrodites: they have two complete reproductive systems, can convert their sex within seconds, and even take turns in fertilizing each other's eggs when coupling. In general, larger size seems to determine which fish more frequently plays the male role.

Even humans, for whom sex seems to be fixed, may have a whole spectrum of feeling and being "feminine" or "masculine." Furthermore, the intensity of feeling one or the other may change during the course of human development, depending on the impact of hormones not only *in utero* but to some extent during postnatal development as well. Environmental challenges and circumstances may also play a very important role. "Masculine" characteristics like taking charge, organizing disparate group members into effective teams, and devising strategies to solve problems and achieve successes can predominate and be fostered among women if there are no males in the social network (such as is the case during a war, for example, when most males are away and women must take on their responsibilities), just as "feminine" tendencies to nurture, rescue, and foster the development of weaker, more dependent individuals may emerge among men when the occasion demands. In fact, drawing skills from both ends of the spectrum is often advantageous. In taking care of patients, I know that sifting and weighing evidence, making swift, informed decisions, and selecting appropriate therapies are essential ingredients for success, but so is a finely honed perception of what any single individual patient requires in terms of comfort and reassurance.

How will new scientific discoveries about the brain, hormones, and biological sex affect you? Researchers are studying the practical application of these discoveries on many issues, but one of the most important is diseases of the central nervous system. What scientists are learning provides doctors with insight into therapeutic maneuvers that will prevent and/or ameliorate those illnesses.

ESTROGEN AND THE BRAIN

Estrogen is not simply a reproductive hormone—it plays a much wider role in the body's growth and maintenance. It is essential to adult men and women for the repair of tissues and organs. In fact, health care experts are considering using hormone replacement therapy to combat some of the changes of aging, including fading memory, for men as well as for women.

Estrogen binds to *receptors* (proteins that "lock onto" a molecule and modulate its activity in a cell) both on the cell membrane and deep within the cell. It has an affinity for specialized receptors inside the *nucleus* (the command center of the cell, which contains our genetic material and regulates the way the cell functions, grows, and repairs itself). There, in combination with other factors, estrogen "turns on" genes that direct the manufacture of new proteins. These new proteins can act within the cell itself or can be exported to influence other cells and tissues.

The varied actions of estrogen throughout the body are explained by specific differences in the estrogen receptors and by the presence or absence of specific co-factors (other proteins that enhance or facilitate the action of estrogen). These co-factors are not only age-specific (present only at one stage of development) but also tissue-specific.

It is estrogen that maintains the brain's plasticity. As we've seen, every piece of new information from the outside world is processed over a unique pathway in the brain, a group of neurons recruited and modified to form a new network. Once established, the new pathway is preserved so that a "memory" of the information is stored in the tissue. It is actually possible to increase the volume of the brain by making new cells to master and retain information. By concentrating on and practicing their particular discipline, for example, musicians can increase the volume of the brain area involved in performing by as much as 25 percent! Estrogen is an essential modulator and facilitator of this process.

Estrogen receptors exist in many parts of the adult brain, and estrogen has specific effects on neurons. It increases the numbers of "spines" on the *dendrites* (the fingerlike projections from the body of a nerve cell). Through these spines neurons communicate with one another by chemical messages released across spaces called *synapses.* These chemicals are called *neurotransmitters.*

Estrogen is also an important regulator of many of the brain's functions. It increases blood flow to the brain and enhances the brain's use of glucose, which provides it with essential energy. In fact, cortical glucose metabolism is 19 percent higher in premenopausal women than in men of the same age.

The Role of Hormonal-Replacement Therapy (HRT) in Memory Preservation and Alzheimer's Disease

Understandably, doctors have become very interested in the importance of estrogen to women who are entering menopause. Studies have shown that rats that are estrogen deficient cannot learn new information; when their brains are examined, their neurons have significantly fewer dendrites than those of estrogen-replete rats. For this reason doctors recommend hormone-replacement therapy (HRT) for postmenopausal women who complain about a loss of memory or a declining ability to think through problems or even to concentrate on a task. (One of my patients calls it "fuzzy thinking.") In perimenopausal and recently menopausal women, estrogen replacement often helps restore the ability to learn and hold on to new data, at least temporarily. A recent review of all existing studies on the impact of estrogen on brain function in postmenopausal women, however, was rather disappointing: the evidence of long-term improvement of women with Alzheimer's disease who were treated with estrogen was not convincing enough for doctors to recommend estrogen for that purpose. Similarly, the results of studies testing whether HRT decreases women's likelihood of developing Alzheimer's disease were contradictory.

Throughout their lives, men have higher estrogen levels than postmenopausal women who are not on HRT. This may account for the differences in the clinical symptoms of men and women who have Alzheimer's: women have more memory impairment and difficulty with language than men, in spite of equally severe deterioration in general cognition. Men with the disease are more likely to have problems with aggressive behavior; women are more likely to be depressed and emotionally labile. B. R. Ott, of Brown University School of Medicine, and his colleagues used single photon emission computed tomography (SPECT) to study blood flow to the brain and found that blood supply to the brain in men and women with Alzheimer's is different. In affected men, blood flow was more frequently depressed in both sides of the brain, while in affected women it was decreased more often only on the left side of the brain.[4] The reasons are unclear but may have to do with gender-specific differences in the distribution and characteristics of estrogen receptors.

"Designer Estrogens" and Their Complications

So-called "designer estrogens" are synthetic hormones that have been specifically manufactured to produce some of estrogen's effects and to avoid others. The synthetically manufactured hormone *tamoxifen*, for example, binds to estrogen receptors in the breast and prevents estrogen from stimulating the production of breast tissue in patients who have developed or are at high risk for breast cancer. Another, *raloxifene*, has a positive impact on bone preservation. While these drugs can be very helpful for many patients, their effects on the brain are not fully understood, so they may introduce other problems into a course of treatment. These "estrogen analogues," as chemists call them, may block estrogen's important maintenance and repair work in the brain. Early study results have been somewhat reassuring: a study of women who were treated with raloxifene for three years showed no demonstrable deterioration in intellectual function.

STROKE IN MEN AND WOMEN

Cerebrovascular accidents (CVAs), more commonly known as strokes, are more frequent in men than in women, but they are more often fatal in women, who tend to be older when they occur. In one study, 25 percent of women who suffered a stroke died as a result, compared with 14 percent of men. Among those who survive, women seem to do worse than men: they have more impaired intellectual function, are less able to care for themselves, and have a higher rate of suicide. In one study of more than 37,000 stroke patients, the suicide rate was twice as high in the female victims, particularly the younger ones.

The risk for stroke is 20 percent higher in women who smoke. Oral contraceptives also increase the risk for stroke, although this risk has decreased with the pill's current lower estrogen dose. Estrogen increases the tendency of blood to clot; its use is particularly dangerous in women who have an increased tendency to coagulate their blood because of abnormalities in their clotting mechanism. Patients with a history of clots in their veins or arteries, particularly those who have had a pulmonary embolus (a clot that circulates in the blood and blocks the blood supply to a certain part of the lung, causing the lung tissue to die), should not use estrogen replacement therapy in any form. The increased risk for a CVA (up to three times higher in oral contraceptive users than in nonusers) is almost entirely due to combining use of the pill with smoking, or to use by women with either high blood pressure or migraine headaches.

DEPRESSION

If hormones produce structural differences in the brain, might they also produce differences in men's and women's emotional behavior? After all, common sense suggests that hormones are important in regulating how we feel: ask any woman about moodiness, irritability, and even "cloudy thinking" just before her menstrual period.

How do hormones regulate mood? While the mechanism is not entirely clear, a growing group of researchers believe that hormones may influence communication between nerve cells. Neurons communicate, as we have seen, through messenger chemicals called neurotransmitters that are secreted by one cell and taken up by another. Several different kinds of chemicals are involved in interneuronal communication, including serotonin, acetylcholine, beta-endorphins, dopamine, and norepinephrine, among others. All of them seem to be involved in the regulation of mood. The amounts and distribution of these neurotransmitters differ in the normal brains of men and women, and aging changes them differently in the two sexes. In animals, estrogen affects the production rate and synaptic concentration of neurotransmitters, but its effects sometimes vary depending on the sex of the animal. In rats, for example, estrogen treatment improves the female's ability to learn but has no effect in males, which respond better to thyroid hormone. In humans, though, estrogen increases the availability, the amount, and the strength of the response of neurons to serotonin; it also increases norepinephrine concentration and the number of receptors for this neurotransmitter in the brain.

Depression can manifest itself quite differently in different people.

Some weep and are outwardly sad, some are cranky and easily fly off the handle, and others are so withdrawn that they sleep most of the time and have very little outward response to the world around them. Depressed women, much more than depressed men, suffer heightened anxiety, or an unreasonable fear of ordinary events (some as mundane as simply leaving the house). Other depressed women endure panic attacks, in which they are paralyzed by a feeling of impending doom and quite literally feel frightened almost to death. Depressed men, on the other hand, are more likely than depressed women to drink excessively or to exhibit violent, abusive behavior.

Do people inherit a tendency to become depressed? Absolutely. Studies of identical twins, even when one has been separated from the other by adoption, show that if one twin has a major depressive illness, the other is more likely to develop it than the average person. The sex of the twin seems to be important as well: fraternal twins of different sexes compared with identical or nonidentical twins of the same sex have a lower incidence of depression. Neuroscientists have not yet pinned down exactly *how* sex influences susceptibility to depression; it is not even certain that the gene(s) is/are carried on the X chromosome.

Depression is undeniably about twice as frequent in women as in men. This difference begins to emerge in midadolescence, and many researchers have suggested that this phenomenon is at least in part cultural, that society's view and treatment of females affects self-esteem and creates feelings of sadness and worthlessness in women. Other data suggest that simply being a biological female is an important factor: the prevalence of depression in women is true in virtually every country of the world (except India*). Certainly social factors affect men and women differently—married men have less depression than married

---

* No one knows for sure why depression in India isn't more frequent in women. Indian women themselves think it is because of the structure of domestic life there, in which several generations of females live together, share domestic responsibilities, and support one another in a tightly knit social fabric. In fact, the incidence of depression in men who are confined to the home and are responsible for child care and domestic chores approaches that of women. The predominance of this illness in women may be more situational than biological!

women, although marriage seems to provide better physical health to both sexes than to people who live alone. Living with children (especially three or more children) doesn't increase the incidence of depression in men, but it does in women—except, interestingly, women in Mediterranean countries. (Some researchers think that this may be because mothers are more highly regarded in those countries than in the rest of the world.) Going to work seems to improve the mood of women who have dependent children; women who work and care for children have less depression than those who stay at home with relatively little adult contact.

Depression and HRT

In women, ovarian steroids (whether naturally occurring or taken as replacement therapy) have a direct impact on mood. Women with severe premenstrual tension find relief from oral contraceptives, which eliminate ovulation. In general, estrogen produces a sense of well-being, while elevated *progesterone* levels (the hormone produced in the second half of the menstrual cycle, from the ovary that has released a mature egg) are correlated with negative moods. This is dramatically apparent when women are given hormones either for birth control or to treat menopause-related conditions. Some of the *progestins* (synthetic hormones) in those medications are more disturbing than others to individual women. The depression and anxiety that accompany the progesterone phase of the cycle in women who use birth control pills can be eliminated or dramatically lessened by using a preparation with a different progestin.

The same sensitivity to progesterone is seen in many post-menopausal women who discontinue HRT because of an unpleasant reaction, not to estrogen (which gives them a sense of vigor and well-being), but to the particular progestin in their prescription, which makes them anxious and weepy. Some women are so sensitive that any progestin is intolerable; for these women, an intrauterine preparation that is not absorbed into the bloodstream is necessary. It is interesting that progestins and tranquilizers bind to the same site on the brain cell;

blocking this site with progestins may increase irritability by making it impossible for calming agents (like diazepam [Valium]) to have an effect. Progestins may also interfere with serotonin-mediated systems. Medications that increase serotonin levels in the synapse (called selective serotonin-reuptake inhibitors or SSRIs; fluoxetine [Prozac] is the best known) are quite effective in treating serious cases of premenstrual tension, called *premenstrual dysphoric disorder* and classified by the American Psychiatric Association as a mental disorder.

Postpartum Depression: When the "Baby Blues" Become Serious

Probably nowhere is the importance of hormones in stabilizing mood more evident than in postpartum depression. Postpartum depression affects one or two women in every thousand births and is related to the abrupt fall in estrogen and progesterone levels that happens within the first day or two of delivery. It is a very serious illness: psychiatric hospital admissions are more likely to happen just after childbirth than at any other time in life. These women are three hundred times more likely than others to become depressed again after delivery of another child. Their babies are often profoundly affected by their illness: they are withdrawn, cannot be comforted, and later in life become depressed themselves. In rare cases the symptoms of postpartum depression are so severe that the mother murders her own children in the throes of a real psychosis, which requires intensive treatment. (In most Western countries, except the United States, the disorder is well recognized as a chief mental illness: women who commit major crimes after delivery are sent for psychiatric treatment rather than to prison, as is the case here.)

Postmenopausal Depression

Estrogen deficiency may also play a role in the depression of post-menopausal women. Use of HRT seems to protect women from the depression that can affect some of them at about ten years after menopause. Other studies have shown that estrogen enhances the effect of SSRIs in relieving depression.

In the elderly estrogen-deficient patient, dementia and depression overlap. Inability to think clearly may actually be due to depression rather than dementia; conversely, about 30 percent of people with progressive dementia also show signs of severe depression. This is not true of younger patients. Whether HRT lessens the likelihood of depression in older women is controversial, but they do respond better to tricyclic antidepressants (such as amitriptyline or Elavil) than to SSRIs. In younger women, on the other hand, SSRIs (like Prozac) are more effective than tricyclics.

STRESS

Whenever you have an unpleasant experience, the resulting stress produces an increase in your adrenal gland's output of *adrenal glucocorticoids*. The levels of these hormones in the bloodstream are controlled by an elaborate feedback mechanism that involves the hippocampal area of the brain, the pituitary, and the adrenal glands themselves. (Like the gonadal steroids, the adrenal glucocorticoids act directly on the brain itself.)

Levels of stress hormones are regulated differently in men and women. When a woman experiences an unpleasant stimulus, estrogen intensifies and prolongs the response of her adrenal glands. Even when young men are given a short course of treatment with estrogen, their response to stress increases! This estrogen link may explain why some girls become more susceptible to stressful conditions at puberty, which is also the age when depression in females begins to be so striking. It may also explain why in many women menopause, when fluctuations in estrogen and progesterone levels diminish, is often accompanied by more emotional stability and a new feeling of well-being. Some experts believe that the interaction between gonadal steroids and the body's response to stress is the reason that diseases associated with increased amounts of emotional pressure (like post-traumatic stress disorder and autoimmune diseases) are more frequent in women than in men.

WHAT DOES THE NEW SCIENCE MEAN FOR YOU?

I'm a fifty-year-old woman and am starting to experience hot flashes, which I know are the beginning of menopause. Recently I've felt more out of sorts than usual and have had problems sleeping. Is there anything to be done about it?

If you are perimenopausal and are having severe mood swings, inability to concentrate, and sleep disturbance, oral contraceptives may provide you with a more stable level of estrogen and improve your symptoms.

My doctor wants to put me on one of the so-called "designer estrogens." Is there anything in particular I should watch out for when taking these?

Don't hesitate to ask your physician to explain any of the drugs she prescribes for you. If you are taking one of these synthesized hormones, be sure to notify her of any unusual side effects, like changes in your mood or your ability to think clearly and effectively or remember new information. It is relatively unlikely but still possible that these medications may be producing more problems for the brain than benefits.

I've got high blood pressure and am taking birth control pills. The little warning that came with the package says that there might be an increased risk of stroke in people like me. Do I need to worry?

You're right—oral contraceptives are slightly chancier in patients who have high blood pressure or migraine headaches and are smokers. Talk with your doctor—these are important factors to consider when deciding which birth control method is right for you.

Sometimes my PMS is so bad that it derails my entire week. I know this isn't unusual and I don't mean to complain, but it's getting exhausting. Ibuprofen takes care of the pain—can anything be done about the emotional roller coaster?

Premenstrual tension, particularly if severe, should prompt you to ask your doctor if an SSRI—a type of antidepressant—will help. Oral contraceptives might also help to stabilize your mood.

I was diagnosed with postpartum depression after both of my children were born; now I'm approaching menopause and am worried that it will return. Also, my daughter is pregnant. I'm wondering if I should mention the possibility of postpartum depression to her, so she'll be better prepared than I was if it happens to her. Are there particular symptoms I should watch for?

The idea that menopause makes you susceptible to depression is not borne out by current information. Instead, menopause often ushers in a period of improved stability, enthusiasm for life, and serenity. But estrogen levels drift downward over a ten-year period following the cessation of menses, which is when older women may experience depression. If this happens to you, you might ask your doctor about HRT rather than an antidepressant, as the hormones may prove to be as effective as an antidepressant. If depression due to estrogen deficiency does become a problem and you elect to try an antidepressant instead of HRT, remember that women are helped more by SSRIs, while depressed men respond better to tricyclic medications like Elavil; ask your doctor how the antidepressant she prescribes for you works.

Your instincts about your daughter are right. Be vigilant after the birth of the baby, and talk with her frequently to get a sense of how she's doing. A brief (two- or three-day) period of the "blues" is very common after delivery, but a lengthy and deepening sense of sadness demands attention from a doctor. Disturbing and repetitive thoughts about harming herself or the new baby are a signal that things are spiraling out of control; she shouldn't be frightened or ashamed of sharing these feelings—they are symptoms of a chemical imbalance that can be treated, not signs of insanity or a criminal mind!

Depression is a labyrinthine illness that can be difficult to recognize, even in oneself. Many people may resist seeking medical attention for a prolonged case of the blues, but it *is* an illness and should be treated like one. Make sure your doctor or therapist discusses practical, "situational" treatments as well as medicinal ones. Getting out of the house more, feeling more useful (such as through paid or volunteer work), and sharing the burden of child care and housework, if you are a mother—all can be just as important as medication in reducing depression. Anxiety and agoraphobia (fear of open places) can be signs of depression in women; in these cases, antidepressants can be more helpful than sedatives (which can often produce a backlash of heightened anxiety or apprehension after wearing off and which are likely to be addictive).

My fourteen-year-old seems to vacillate between personalities: the sweet, confident child that she was and a tearful young woman with an acrid tongue. My husband feels that we should just leave her alone, but I'd like to do what I can for her, though she often barely acknowledges me.

Adolescence can be a very difficult time. Adolescent girls and their parents should bear in mind that changing hormone levels can bring about dramatic and very real challenges to self-confidence. Talking, emotional support, and seeking the help of counselors can be very helpful in working out some of these feelings before they become overwhelming for her and for the family.

CHAPTER 3

Drug Metabolism

_____

S O MANY THINGS are involved in the body's processing of a medication that no doctor should dismiss out of hand a patient's report of an unusual reaction. It's a tricky task to weigh one's knowledge against a situation that confounds it, but one of the biggest mistakes physicians can make is to say, "I've never heard of this problem, and I can't explain it; *ergo,* the patient must be crazy / unreliable / just plain mistaken."

I've prescribed a certain medication for my patient Jane, who now tells me she can't stand even the tiniest dose of it. I've ordered the liquid form of the drug, used for children, so she can begin with only a few drops. But even that makes her intolerably sleepy. My patient Harry, on the other hand, swallows a much larger dose of the same medication and tells me he feels nothing at all. He has to take twice the usual dose before he reports an effect. Jane isn't hysterical; she's not imagining that she's so sensitive. But Harry's not hysterical either. So it's up to me to try to discover what's causing the two of them to react so differently to the same drug.

The answer seems simple enough; Jane's and Harry's weight and body composition obviously differ. (Jane weighs about 125 pounds and Harry 165.) But the difference in their doses was huge, more than enough to compensate for the disparity in size. My most important clue in this case may actually be the gender difference itself. Clinical trials of this particular medication, which worked out the doses that would be both safe and effective for patients, were conducted only in men. Everyone involved in testing—and approving the drug for use— assumed that data from men would be the same in women. Let's take a look at why that isn't necessarily so.

PHARMACOKINETICS: HOW THE BODY PROCESSES DRUGS

Most people believe that the medications they take will work the way the label or the doctor tells them they will: aspirin will relieve a headache, antibiotics will cure an infection, and a sleeping pill will produce a peaceful night. In reality, many things determine how your body will react to a medicine—even something as simple as the way you take the drug into your body. For example, swallowing a pill generally produces a slower and less reliable effect than injecting a drug directly into the bloodstream. Most of the time people don't need to feel the effects of a medicine urgently enough to warrant the extra fuss and discomfort of an injection, but in more critical situations, when every second counts, an injection can literally be a lifesaver.

How the body absorbs a medicine, distributes it in the tissues, and then eliminates it when it's no longer useful is called its *pharmacokinetics*. The pharmacokinetics of a drug depend on many factors. how completely and how rapidly it is absorbed, its distribution in the body (a fat-soluble drug, for example, will concentrate in areas that are rich in fat), how much of it binds to carrier-proteins in the blood, and how efficiently the liver breaks it down and presents the remnants to the kidney or the lung so they can be eliminated from the body.

Differences in the pharmacokinetics of a given drug can result from variations in individual circumstances, or they may be due to more general characteristics, including the patient's sex. The drug may interact with other drugs the person is taking. The acid level in his stomach, the enzymes in her gastrointestinal tract, his genetic makeup, her inherited susceptibilities and conditions, and his body composition (fat or muscle) may all affect a drug's pharmacokinetics. Some physical conditions or illnesses (like diabetes) have a significant impact on the body's ability to metabolize drugs. Many differences in pharmacokinetics are related, either directly or indirectly, to the sex of the patient. But before we explore a few of the most important differences in the ways males and females process drugs, let's get a quick overview of pharmacokinetics, identifying notable gender-specific characteristics along the way.

Absorption: How a Drug Gets from Your Mouth into Your Tissues

If you take a medicine by mouth, its effect on you will depend on how well your stomach or intestines can absorb it and deliver it to the bloodstream, so it can be carried to the tissue where it will do its job. Sometimes food or other medications combine with a drug or even destroy it before it has a chance to be absorbed. Iron and the aluminum in antacids, for example, combine with tetracyclines (a kind of antibiotic) in the stomach so that the tetracyclines can't cross the intestinal wall and get into the bloodstream. Other medications need stomach acid in order to dissolve, so if you take them with a medicine that blocks acid production (like ranitidine [Zantac] or omeprazole [Prilosec]), they can't be absorbed. For example, taking estrogen by mouth after a meal, when acid production is at a maximum, helps absorption.

Some drugs leave the intestine and enter the bloodstream differently in males and females. Girls absorb iron, for example, more easily than boys, perhaps explaining why iron-deficiency anemias are more common in eleven-to-fifteen-year-old boys than in girls of the same age. Our gastrointestinal tracts behave differently: women have less acid in the stomach and slower emptying times than men—except in the middle of the menstrual cycle, when the speed of gastric emptying increases. This factor would lengthen the amount of time a drug stayed in a female stomach and perhaps increase its effects.

Women and men clearly metabolize alcohol differently, *depending on how it enters the body*. When I was an intern at Bellevue Hospital in New York, I learned that one of the cheapest and most effective ways to prevent DTs (delirium tremens) in alcoholic patients is to give them, intravenously, a slow drip of alcohol, then gradually lessen it to prevent withdrawal. The same dose was effective for both sexes: women and men have exactly the same levels of blood alcohol if it is given by vein. But if alcohol is taken by mouth, women's blood levels are higher than those of men. Females have only about one-fifth as much of the enzyme that breaks down alcohol (alcohol dehydrogenase) in their stomachs as males, so women literally get more effect from alcohol, ounce for ounce, than do men (as long as they drink it!).

Researchers haven't studied these phenomena extensively, but differences such as these clearly provide valuable clues for ways to gender-specialize the treatment of disease.

How the Drug Gets to the Right Place in Your Body

Once a medication is absorbed, what happens to it? It is carried in the liquid part of the blood (called *serum*), until it reaches the tissues on which it will act. Along the way some of the drug may combine with a special carrier or *binding protein* in the serum. In general, the body can use only the free form of the medicine, so protein binding reduces the usable and available amount. Estrogen lowers the concentration of one binding protein (alpha$_4$ acid glycoprotein). The concentrations of another class of binding proteins (the lipoproteins) can vary with the sex of the individual, as can specific carriers like sex-hormone-binding globulin or corticosteroid-binding globulin. Some medicines may travel alone, without the help of a carrier at all.

Doctors and pharmacists must be very careful about drug interactions, in part because several medicines may compete for the same binding protein. (Oral contraceptives, for example, often compete for the same carriers used by common medications.) The amount of a drug that is bound affects the dose that the patient needs in order to have an effect. As if all this weren't complicated enough, many other things also affect the amount of drug bound to serum proteins: age, smoking, and obesity. Even daily cyclical changes in the affinity between the drug and its binding proteins can affect the process! (This might be the reason your physician asks you to take your medicine before sleep instead of in the morning, for example.)

Once a drug is on its way, how does it "know" which tissues or cells to act on? How does the aspirin you are taking for your headache know where it has to go to reduce your pain? The answer lies in *receptors*, the specialized proteins in cell membranes that we discussed in Chapter 2. These docking sites are specially tailored for molecules of the drug you take in. In a sense, they are uniquely structured "locks" that only the drug molecule "key" can fit into and open. Once it enters and opens the receptors, the drug actually changes a cell's function and produces the desired effect, which can be as monumental as killing the cell or bacterium (as in the case of a cancer drug or an antibiotic) or as simple as changing some of the steps in the cell's life process so that it works more efficiently. (The heart medicine digitalis, for example, increases cardiac cells' ability to contract.) If the tissue through which the medicine is traveling has no receptor, the drug has no effect. Designing a new drug involves making molecules that will fit into receptors on bacteria and on the cells of our own tissue so effectively that the medication will affect that target cell's metabolism with as few unwanted side effects as possible.

The time a medicine takes to have an effect can vary dramatically. Some drugs, like phenytoin (Dilantin), commonly used to control seizures, reach their receptor sites almost immediately. Others, like digitalis, can take up to eight hours to have an effect, because binding to receptors and the consequent changes in the heart cells' metabolism take place so slowly.

How Your Body Gets Rid of a Drug

It's important for your body to be able to eliminate a drug once it is no longer needed. How fast a drug is broken down and excreted is one of the most important indicators of how long it will work, and how intensely.

The rate of kidney function determines how quickly a drug is eliminated from the body and therefore how long the patient feels its effects. Kidney function is indirectly affected by gender because, in general, the rate at which the kidneys filter and purify the blood (called the glomerular filtration rate, or GFR) is more rapid in people with higher body weights. On average, women's filtration rates are lower than men's, except during pregnancy, when GFR increases. Other drugs, however, are cleared faster by the premenopausal woman's kidneys, like the pain medication alfentanil. The difference in filtration rates disappears with age, and after fifty relatively rapid clearance in women is no longer an issue.

The Body's Sanitation Department: The P450 System

The sanitation functions of the liver and intestinal tract are complicated but are worth a quick overview.

The liver and the intestinal tract contain a family of proteins or enzymes called the *cytochrome P450 system,* which breaks up drug molecules and changes their configuration so they can be absorbed and ultimately excreted by the kidneys. The most important members of the family are the CYP 3A4 enzymes, which account for as much as 60 percent of drug metabolism. (This includes the metabolism of sex hormones, both our own naturally produced ones and those used for replacement therapy or birth control.) Important siblings of CYP 3A4 are the CYP 1A enzymes, which metabolize acetaminophen (Tylenol), theophylline, tamoxifen, and warfarin (Coumadin). Caffeine-containing beverages and smoking affect the action of the CYP 3A4 subfamily on medications. CYP 2C enzymes control the metabolism of diazepam (Valium) and phenytoin (Dilantin). The CYP 2D6 subfamily processes many of the drugs prescribed for mood and mental disorders like haloperidol (Haldol), clozapine, amitriptyline (Elavil), imipramine (Tofranil), nortriptyline, and the beta-blockers propranolol and timolol, which are used to treat heart patients and people with high blood pressure.

Some medicines, including phenobarbital, Dilantin, and alcohol itself actually stimulate the production of these various enzymes in the liver cell. These medications (called inducing drugs) will increase the rates at which other drugs are metabolized, lessening their efficacy. Inducing drugs can reduce the concentrations of many medications in the body, including steroids, anticoagulants like warfarin (Coumadin), oral contraceptives, and some antibiotics. Genetics also affects how quickly an individual will metabolize a drug, by influencing the number of enzymes an individual has. This may affect the degree to which a person is able to metabolize a medication by tenfold or more.

WHY MEN AND WOMEN RESPOND DIFFERENTLY TO MEDICINES

Gender Differences in Pharmacokinetics: The P450 System

That the type, concentration, and intensity of activity of P450 enzymes differ between men and women is a significant part of the reason that men and women respond differently to some medications: *they metabolize them differently.* Sex-specific patterns of drug metabolism, scientists believe, are due to the different ways males and females secrete growth hormone, which are determined during brain development. The pattern in males, established by testosterone, consists of bursts of growth hormone alternating with periods of low hormone production. Females, by contrast, produce growth hormone at a constant rate. Somatostatin, a chemical produced in the brain, inhibits growth hormone production and "feminizes" the pattern of drug metabolism in males. Insulin has important stabilizing effects on growth hormone, and as a result diabetics, some of whom suffer from lack of insulin, often have major problems with drug metabolism; insulin treatment often returns these people to normal.

Recent animal studies have shown us a startling characteristic of the P450 system: the thin layer of fat in which the enzymes themselves are embedded within the liver cell is itself different in males and females. In fact, if the enzymes from a male are isolated and embedded in a female lipid layer, the pattern of drug metabolism is feminized. This kind of discovery points research in humans in important new directions.

What Are Some Drugs That Men and Women Metabolize Differently?

Women have a more active CYP 3A4 system than men, which is particularly important because this group of enzymes is responsible for the metabolism of up to 60 percent of all drugs; the CYP 3A4 system has up to 40 percent more activity in women than in men. (Scientists attribute these differences to women's higher levels of progesterone, since in laboratory studies progesterone activates this system.) Women clear from their system several medications metabolized by the CYP 3A4 system much faster than men do. Among these are an antibiotic (erythromycin), prednisolone (a steroid), verapamil (a calcium channel blocker used in heart patients and in people with hypertension; women had more rapid heart rates after receiving the drug than did men), and diazepam (Valium).

The Effect of Hormones on Drug Metabolism

Until 1993 women of childbearing age were specifically excluded from research that tested new drugs. This exclusion was not so much mali-cious as a humanitarian, as an effort to protect women and developing fetuses from damage. The assumption (read: hope) was that the differences between men and women were so minimal that the safety and efficacy data obtained in men would also apply to women. But as scientists have learned more about women's unique physiology, they have come to understand the gravity of this error. In some instances, drugs that were safe for men were dangerous and even deadly for women. A great deal of research must still be done to evaluate the safety and effects of many drugs in women.

Estrogen and progesterone are metabolized by the P450 system, so women might be expected to metabolize the medicines that are processed in that system differently from men. Women taking certain medications must be watched (and must watch themselves) very carefully for any changes in the drugs' side effects or any loss of efficacy. For example, some of the antifungal drugs, if given for a long period of time, might require a woman to take a lower dose of estrogen. On the other hand, some medications actually induce the production and impact the activity of some of the components of the P450 system, like phenytoin (Dilantin) or rifampin (a medication used to treat tuberculosis). Women taking such medications might need to boost their dose of estrogen to maintain the benefit of HRT.

Another consideration for women is that their hormone shifts may have a significant impact on the way they process drugs, even though everything else (the dose, the time of day, the relationship to meals) remains the same. As we have discussed, estrogen levels rise during the first half of the menstrual cycle, and peak at about midcycle. After ovulation, progesterone levels begin to rise, and are highest just before menses (when, in contrast, estrogen levels are quite low). Sometimes women with epilepsy have seizures just before or during the first part of the menstrual period: this *catamenial epilepsy* is probably due to a progesterone-mediated increase in CYP 3A4 activity, which metabolizes Dilantin and other antiepileptic drugs. The same thing happens in epileptic women's pregnancies for the same reason; a woman whose seizures were well controlled before her pregnancy may need her dosage increased. Methylprednisolone (a drug often used to treat severe asthma or allergic attacks) is metabolized differently at different phases of the menstrual cycle: estrogen seems to make women more sensitive to the medication, but it also causes the drug to be metabolized more quickly, so there is no need to change the dose of the drug as a function of the menstrual cycle—these two effects seem to cancel each other out!

Six diseases seem to intensify in a significant proportion of women who have them premenstrually: asthma, arthritis, migraine headaches, diabetes, depression, and epilepsy. If a woman who has one of these illnesses tracks her symptoms and discovers changes premenstrually, she should be particularly careful about avoiding triggering factors during her vulnerable periods. Her usual medication doses might have to be increased during these times, or her ovulation suppressed with oral contraceptives.

Menopause might also be expected to have an impact on how women process medications; dosage requirements and even reactions to the drugs might change because of changes in the activity of the P450 system when ovarian hormone production falls off. Unfortunately, scientists have very little data yet about the impact of menopause on drug metabolism and even less about the changes that might occur as a result of HRT.

Other complicating factors specific to gender don't involve the liver. Women on the anticoagulant drug warfarin (Coumadin) may have to carefully monitor their reactions to estrogen. Estrogen and Coumadin compete to bind to the same plasma protein, so estrogen might diminish Coumadin binding, freeing more of it to produce more marked anticoagulation. This may, though, be balanced by estrogen's natural tendency to make women clot more easily. Premenopausal women, women on oral contraceptives, and postmenopausal women on HRT may have to be watched more carefully than other patients on anticoagulation therapy and may require more frequent laboratory testing to find the ideal dose of both Coumadin and estrogen.

DRUG ABUSE

How Do Addictive Drugs Work?

Scientists now know the precise location of receptors for every major drug that patients abuse and precisely how each of them acts on the brain. All have one thing in common: they all cause the release of the neurotransmitter *dopamine* in a system of neuronal connections called the *reward pathway* (or *VTA-NA system*), a feedback system that controls feelings of well-being and satisfaction. It is dopamine that produces the positive experience addicts seek.

Three major classes of drugs can affect the function of the VTA-NA system in different ways.

• *Stimulants* (like cocaine, nicotine, and amphetamines) increase the concentration of dopamine in the synapses.

• *Sedatives* (like alcohol, benzodiazepines [Valium], and barbiturates) depress arousal by increasing the action of a sedating neurotransmitter called GABA, which lowers the excitability of neurons in the VTA-NA system.

• *Opiates* (like heroin and morphine) work on portions of the VTA-NA system to produce euphoria and an enhanced sense of well-being. But they also change the reactivity of stimulating neurons that use norepinephrine as a transmitter; these are under constant inhibition in normal brains, but chronic use of opiates makes them hypersensitive, and when opiates are stopped, a tremendous surge of stimulating chemicals produces a withdrawal syndrome.

Drug Addiction in Men and Women

There are some striking differences in the way men and women use addictive substances.

- Twenty-two percent more men than women abuse illicit drugs, but women are more at risk of becoming dependent on prescribed medications like Valium, perhaps because of their higher susceptibility to anxiety.
- The progression from alcohol or nicotine abuse (the first drugs used in the addiction cycle by both sexes) to illicit substances is well described. For men, alcohol alone precedes the use of other drugs, but for women, cigarettes are also important.
- The first illicit drug that both men and women try is marijuana.
- For women, the rate of childbearing increases when there is a high rate of illicit drug use.
- Tobacco addiction is somewhat different between the sexes. Women seem to struggle with it more than men, perhaps because in women, smoking is less likely to be related strictly to dependence on nicotine, as it seems to be in men. Women may also value the sensory and social factors in smoking, and treatment with nicotine substitutes works less well for them than for men. Women have more difficulty quitting, gain more weight, and experience more severe withdrawal symptoms than men do.
- Another sex-specific vulnerability to nicotine may be established in the womb: daughters *(but not sons)* of women who smoked during pregnancy are four times more likely to begin smoking during adolescence than the daughters of women who didn't smoke during pregnancy. Nicotine reaches the fetus across the placental barrier (which is how the mother's body protects the fetus from dangerous substances) and may well selectively affect the developing brain of the female fetus.

• Alcohol, cocaine, opiates, and other addictive drugs disrupt the menstrual cycle and decrease women's fertility.

• Younger women's higher estrogen levels may protect them against some of the vasoconstrictive effects of cocaine in the brain and heart that produce the strokes and cardiac arrhythmias seen in addicted men.

• Women have lower levels of cocaine in their blood and a blunted response to it during or after the middle of their cycle; men, on the other hand, have a consistent response to cocaine.

• Women seem to return to drug use after trying to quit as a consequence of bad emotional experiences and feelings, but men describe quite positive emotional states just prior to relapse: "If high feels good, higher will feel better!" On the other hand, women seem to relapse less frequently than men, possibly because they use group counseling more often and more effectively.

PSYCHOTROPIC MEDICATIONS IN MEN AND WOMEN

Almost anyone who has been treated for depression with medicine knows that physicians often have to find the right drug through trial and error. Sometimes the first or second choice produces intolerable side effects or has little or no effect, while another works beautifully to restore the patient to a more normal state. A drug that seems to have worked well for a long period of time may suddenly stop working, and the physician must either change the dose or choose an entirely different medication. These powerful and relatively new chemicals that change mood and correct psychosis are called *psychotropic medications*. While much of our information about them is still quite rudimentary, careful observation has told us enough to make some general statements about gender differences in response to these drugs.

Young women seem more sensitive to the effects of psychotropic medications; even when the doses are corrected for body size, women show a more pronounced response, including being more likely to suffer unpleasant or unwanted side effects than men. While these responses may be due to the effect of estrogen on the brain, they may also be attributed to differences in the pharmacokinetics of the drugs that we don't yet appreciate. Men seem to process and excrete at least one of the drugs used to treat schizophrenia (fluphenazine) more rapidly than do women.

Men with anxiety attacks respond better to imipramine (Tofranil) than do women. Tricyclic antidepressants like Elavil are very effective in treating depressed men with panic attacks, but women with the same disorders respond better to monoamine oxidase inhibitors like tranylcypromine (Parnate). One antidepressant, paroxetine (Paxil), works by prolonging the time serotonin remains at the synapse between nerve cells; it is more effective in women. This seems to be due to a fundamental difference in the way brain cells bind to serotonin. Serotonin receptors on cells called platelets circulate in the blood, and men's platelets have fewer binding sites for serotonin than do those of women.

DO DOCTORS KNOW HOW TO PRESCRIBE FOR MENSTRUATING OR PREGNANT WOMEN?

Because drug trials have so rarely included premenopausal women, doctors know very little about the impact of naturally cycling hormones on pharmacokinetics and pharmacodynamics. Researchers have observed a few individual medicines in very small numbers of women but usually for only one or two cycles at the most. To confuse the issue, scientists often divide up the menstrual cycle differently, into anywhere from two to five stages. Many don't use failsafe parameters to measure when—or even whether—ovulation has occurred. This, as you might imagine, makes it rather difficult to determine what if any effects the monthly cycle has on drug absorption, metabolization, side effects, and efficacy. Here as elsewhere we need meaningful numbers of observations in meaningful numbers of women studied with generally-agreed-upon methodologies. For now, perhaps the best you can do as an individual is to carefully note any differences in your response to the medicines you're taking (especially at the beginning of a new treatment) over the course of at least three or four menstrual cycles, and let your doctor know about them. You could do the same for courses of birth control pills and HRT (particularly if you have begun it recently and if you take estrogen and progesterone in a cyclic rather than a concurrent fashion).

WHAT DO WE *REALLY* KNOW ABOUT USING NEW DRUGS IN WOMEN?

The Food and Drug Administration has developed one of the most careful procedures in the world to determine whether a new medicine is safe and effective. Consequently the pharmaceutical industry has to meet extensive requirements when securing permission to market a new drug.

Before the FDA will approve any new drug, the manufacturer must successfully negotiate several distinct steps:

- Preclinical study: This is the first stage of testing and is usually performed in animals. The preclinical study is designed to determine the impact of the drug, its safety (at least in the model being tested), how the body prepares it for activity (its pharmacokinetics), and finally how it actually works (its pharmacodynamics).
- Phase I: The drug is tested in 20 to 80 human volunteers; the right doses are worked out, and the human pharmacokinetics and pharmacodynamics are mapped.
- Phase II: A larger group of very closely watched patients (100 to 200), people who have the condition for which the medication was designed, are tested. The safety and effectiveness of the drug is tested, and the proper dosage is refined. Any adverse reactions are carefully noted and studied.
- Phase III: This much larger trial involves sometimes thousands of patients. The same parameters are tested as in phase II; in fact, in some cases phase III studies can be mounted at the same time as phase II investigations.

• Phase IV: After the drug has been approved, postmarketing surveillance monitors what happens to patients using the drug for longer
periods of time.

Many of the drugs we use every day were tested almost exclusively
in men. Women were included in about half of the studies before 1988,
when FDA guidelines grew more demanding, but there were seldom
enough of them to allow researchers to draw any firm conclusions about
gender differences. Moreover, the women included in studies were
almost invariably postmenopausal and hence were not subject to cyclic
variations in their hormones. Many women (and the physicians who
cared for them) feared that an untested medication might affect their
ability to bear children or even their unborn children. This attitude persists today. Unless a young woman is very ill, she is usually reluctant to
volunteer to be part of a clinical trial of a new drug. The company making and testing the medicine is equally reluctant to accept her into the
study: as one pharmaceutical company executive commented, "It will
take only one more thalidomide disaster to set us back two decades in
the progress we've made in including premenopausal women in clinical
trials." As a result, most of what we know about women (and children,
for that matter) and a given medication comes from observations made
after they are given the drug during the course of an illness.

In 1988 the FDA mandated that drugs intended for women had to
be tested in women before they could be approved for distribution and
sale. This requirement signaled a significant change in the procedure
for new drug development and approval. It was very slowly imple-
mented, however, and in 1993 the FDA promulgated specific guidelines for evaluating gender differences in how drugs were to be tested.
Compliance with the new demand has been slow and imperfect, but at
the present time almost all new drug applications include at least pre-
liminary data from both sexes.

Scientists still have a way to go: recent analysis has shown gender
differences as large as 50 percent in 28 percent of the unpublished
data.[1] To put it another way, in over a quarter of the data coming from
drug trials researchers are currently conducting, the differences in values are as large as twofold between men and women.

It is not enough to generate the numbers; doctors and scientists must understand them and use them judiciously. To safeguard women adequately, we have to be much more vigilant not only in scrutinizing initial data but in monitoring all phases of clinical testing—and as Janice Schwartz, of Northwestern University Medical School, has suggested in her recent review of the system, we are not doing a very good job for the female patient.[2] For example, in two recently released medications, cerivastatin (used to lower dangerously high levels of serum cholesterol) and mibefradil (used to treat angina), the data from testing showed gender-specific effects that were largely disregarded, to the detriment of the women who were given the drugs. In the case of cerivastatin, the concentrations in women were 12 percent higher than in men after a single dose, and females, especially the elderly, were more likely to have muscle destruction as a side effect. Nonetheless the drug was not only approved for release but *had to be withdrawn from the market after approval and was in fact prompt_withdrawn from the market after approval and was in fact general_publication* because of the unacceptably high incidence of fatal muscle destruction in treated women. The same scenario was true of mibefradil, which was removed from the market for the same reasons.

Here are what Janice Schwartz lists as vitally important points for patients and their physicians to consider in prescribing medications:

• Sex-specific information on drugs approved before the mid-1990s may not exist.

• Some sex-specific data ought to be available on drugs tested after 1993, when data were analyzed according to gender.

• The number of women involved in pre-release testing may not be sufficient to guarantee safety and efficacy or even proper dosing in women.

• Very few pregnant women have been involved in drug testing.

• Physicians must be very alert to any untoward event or unanticipated reaction to a medication, particularly in female patients.

These guidelines are just a start. Doctors and patients must begin to think differently about the entire process, and we can only do that if we are armed with the facts.

WHAT DOES THE NEW SCIENCE MEAN FOR YOU?

My doctor recently prescribed atorvastatin (Lipitor) to correct my high cholesterol. As a woman, what should I know about the new class of medications called the statins?

The statins, which interfere with cholesterol synthesis in the liver and improve the power of liver cells to remove harmful low-density lipoprotein (LDL) from the bloodstream, are important new additions to the drugs that prevent and mitigate the ravages of coronary artery disease. The statins produce greater reductions in "bad" cholesterol levels at the same time as they raise the level of "good" cholesterol or high-density lipoprotein (HDL, the lipoprotein most important for protection from coronary artery disease in women). This is particularly important because low HDL (below 35) is a more serious risk factor for women than for men. In the past, we had only estrogen and niacin as agents to increase HDL levels; both of them can have important and sometimes unacceptable side effects.

Will a statin be efficacious and safe for you as a woman? On the whole, these drugs work well, have few negative side effects, and are the most useful agents we've ever had to correct high levels of LDL and improve levels of HDL.

- The statins lower cholesterol more and are better tolerated than other available agents.
- Several of the large trials of the statins included significant numbers of women and proved that women had the same level of benefit from their use as did men.
- Some data suggest that patients who use statin drugs are *less likely to have fractures* than patients who do not use them.
- No significant interaction of the statins with oral contraceptives or HRT has been observed. Some data suggest that estrogen augments the effect of statins.
- Women over sixty may be more likely to suffer muscle pain than younger women or men on these medications. Report this prob-

lem to your physician immediately, and follow her recommendations for monitoring your condition with blood testing during the course of your therapy very carefully.

Almost every time I have my menstrual period, I have an epileptic seizure. My doctor tells me it's because I'm more tense and emotional at this time. Is he right?

No, he's unaware of the fact that the higher progesterone levels of the premenstrual period accelerate the metabolism of Dilantin. He should increase your Dilantin dosage in the days just before your menstrual period. This is the catamenial epilepsy we discussed earlier in the chapter.

I take Coumadin, an anticoagulant drug, for my chronic atrial fibrillation. I've just been put on oral contraceptives and find that it's harder to stabilize the daily dose of Coumadin I need. Is there a connection?

Yes. Coumadin and estrogen compete to bind on the same sites on proteins in the serum (the liquid part of the blood). You may need to lower your dose of Coumadin to compensate for this.

My husband took one of my diazepam (Valium) pills the other day and slept all night. I find that the same pill simply doesn't sedate me that long: I often awaken anyway at three in the morning. Why the difference?

You may need more frequent doses of Valium to get the same effect as your husband. Women clear Valium from their system more quickly than men because the enzyme system in the liver that metabolizes it is 40 percent more active in women!

I've recently been put on a medicine to control my irregular pulse. Sometimes I think I'm worse with the medicine than without it: the extra beats seem more frequent and sometimes I actually feel as though I'm going to faint. What's wrong? Is this just anxiety, or is something really wrong?

Something may really be wrong: women are more likely to develop paradoxical *increases* in disturbances in their heart rhythm with the very drugs that were chosen to reduce them because they have been shown in clinical trials to eliminate extra beats and stabilize the heart. The basic normal function of women's hearts is different enough from men's to make a significant number of females vulnerable to this unusual but potentially lethal effect of the medication. Report these symptoms at once to your doctor; if he dismisses them, ask to be referred to a cardiologist who is aware of this gender-specific vulnerability.

My son has been given amitriptyline (Elavil) for his anxiety attacks. I thought fluoxetine (Prozac) was a newer and better drug. Why did his doctor choose the older medication?

Anxiety in men responds better to the tricyclic drugs like Elavil, while women are more successful with the selective serotonin-reuptake inhibitors (SSRIs) like Prozac. Women may have more abundant serotonin receptors on the neurons in their central nervous system than men, and men may require a larger dose of an SSRI than a woman to achieve the same relief from anxiety.

I get wonderful relief from my pain medication sometimes but much less at others. What could be the reason?

Try noting the phase of your menstrual cycle when you have less than the usual effect. Progesterone, which is higher in the second half of your cycle, inhibits the absorption of some medicines in the stomach and slows down the transit time of medicine (and everything else you swallow) through your intestinal tract. If this pattern becomes apparent, you may need to tailor the dose of your painkiller depending on the phase of your cycle.

I can't tolerate the medicine my doctor has just prescribed: it nauseates me and makes me feel faint, even when I take half of what she's prescribed. She

says she's never heard of that and tells me I'm just depressed and anxious.
Am I crazy, or is there a reason for my complaints?

There may well be a reason for your unusual reaction to the drug, and the fact that your doctor has never heard of it doesn't make you crazy. Rather, your doctor should report your experience to the manufacturer, as this may be one of the drugs that haven't been satisfactorily studied in women. They need all the feedback they can get! Ask your doctor to adjust your dosage until your side effects are relieved.

CHAPTER 4

The Gastrointestinal Tract

D URING MY FIRST year in medical school, my Viennese professor opened his lecture on the gastrointestinal tract with an
image so vivid that I never forgot it. He observed that we are
essentially elaborate doughnuts, that the gastrointestinal tract, running
through our bodies from mouth to anus, is simply an empty space in
the middle of our otherwise solid selves. Thankfully, the situation turns
out to be a bit more complicated than that. The gastrointestinal system
is a specialized organ of incredible complexity and competence. Not
only does it transform our food into the fuel and building components
we need for tissue repair and maintenance, it contains an intricate system of neurons that some scientists have dubbed our "second brain,"
which communicates constantly with the "first" brain inside the skull;
so what's happening in the world around us can literally have gut-
wrenching consequences. Much as the skin provides external protection, the gut protects us on the inside from the innumerable foreign
substances and organisms that would otherwise invade and damage the
body. Finally, it ushers what we don't need out of the body with
remarkable efficiency, ensuring that the fluids and salts on which our
tissues depend aren't lost in the process.

Unfortunately, scientists have more questions than answers about
the gender-specific characteristics of the gastrointestinal tract, but the
things we do understand have pointed our research in valuable direc-

tions. We know that food takes longer to pass through a woman's GI tract than through a man's; that the hormonal shifts of the menstrual cycle and pregnancy affect gastrointestinal *motility* (the contractions of the gut that move food along); that bile from a woman's liver is different from bile from a man's (which helps explain the higher incidence of gallstones in women than in men); and that up to six times as many women as men suffer from a painful and in many cases debilitating illness called *irritable bowel syndrome* (IBS). Many women who suffer from gastrointestinal disruptions (such as diarrhea while menstruating and IBS) or from more serious illnesses that inflame and destroy the lining of the intestine (like Crohn's disease and ulcerative colitis) will benefit enormously from this research. It will especially help those whose problems have gone largely untreated or been assigned the unhelpful diagnosis of "functional" bowel disease (often meaning an aberration that one must just endure, since doctors don't really understand it and can't cure it).

For now, though, it will be helpful to survey the newest discoveries, disparate though they are, that shed new light on the gender specificity of many of the parts and disorders of the digestive system.

ELEMENTS OF THE DIGESTIVE SYSTEM AND THEIR RELATED AILMENTS

Saliva

The moment you open your mouth to eat, the food meets a gender-specific environment: your saliva.

Probably the least vaunted member of the digestive system, saliva nonetheless plays a complicated role: it maintains the proper balance of acid, sugar, and digestive enzymes to prepare food for digestion; disposes of hostile invaders (such as unwanted bacteria); and lubricates the mouth for fluent speech. Adequate amounts of saliva and high oxygen content keep down the bacterial growth in your mouth. (The reason you have bad breath on awakening is because salivary flow rates drop during sleep and mouth bacteria deplete the available oxygen during sleep.)

Saliva is also useful because it reflects events in the rest of the body. In healthy people, the sugar and electrolyte content of saliva varies during the course of a day in a predictable cycle. (Electrolytes are electrically charged ions, like sodium, potassium, and calcium.) These variations also occur during women's monthly cycle. During menstruation, for example, the glucose content of saliva increases three- to ninefold. (Bacteria will profit from the increased concentration of sugar in the saliva; so women should probably be particularly scrupulous about brushing and flossing during their menstrual periods, to combat gum infection and tooth decay.) During ovulation, on the other hand, calcium and sodium levels in saliva go down and that of potassium increases. Some of the enzymes that help to break down food (salivary peroxidases) are also more active during ovulation, which may be the body's way of preparing nutrients for a new fetus that might soon appear on the scene.

Because hormone concentrations are detectable in saliva, it is being used more and more to test patients for the presence of specific diseases and conditions. For example, determining the progesterone concentration in saliva is an excellent way to find out whether a woman is ovulating. (In fact, only when researchers started testing saliva for this reason did they learn that even women who menstruate regularly do not necessarily ovulate predictably.) A side effect of oral contraceptives is that they help maintain optimal acid content in saliva. (A high acid concentration actually helps prevent bad breath because it lowers the amount of bacteria in the mouth.) Postmenopausal HRT, on the other hand, appears not to influence salivary gland function.

Ultimately, I believe, saliva may provide us with important clues about both the normal and the pathological functioning of the body, for both sexes. Men have a higher resting and food-stimulated flow rate of saliva than women, for example, but we don't yet know exactly why. Male saliva has higher yeast content, although again we don't know why. An individual's health has a big impact on the composition and production of saliva: depressed patients of both sexes have lower salivary flow rates, even when medication and lack of appetite are taken into consideration. The same is true of diabetic patients, unless their blood sugar is well controlled. As research continues to unlock its secrets, saliva will play a growing role as a diagnostic tool.

The Esophagus

The esophagus is the short tube that contracts when you swallow, pushing swallowed food forward into your stomach. A few aspects of its normal function are gender specific. The esophagus is shorter in women than in men, and distending it causes women more pain (which seems true of much of the gastrointestinal tract). Its contractions are more frequent and more forceful in women than in men, producing symptoms that can mimic the chest pains associated with a heart attack, an important point for an examining physician to consider.

The lower end of the esophagus is protected from backflow of stomach acid and food by a ring of muscle; when this ring isn't functioning properly, the stomach's contents regurgitate into the lower portion of the esophagus, a condition called *gastroesophageal reflux disease* (GERD). This acid-laden food causes a burning discomfort and even painful spasms of the esophagus itself, which can be quite troublesome. Lying down often makes the problem worse; sometimes patients wake up choking and actually inhale the regurgitated food; some literally can't breathe because of a reactive spasm of the upper airway. Asthma and even pneumonia can result. A subtler sign of GERD is a persistent cough. Often patients go through several bronchoscopies (examinations of their airways under anesthesia) to look for cancer, when in fact their problem is an airway irritated by repeated exposure to corrosive stomach acid.

While GERD is marginally more common in women (3.18 percent versus 2.94 percent in men), in whom symptoms can be more bothersome, the disease is actually more serious in men. In fact, men produce more stomach acid and have more acid reflux even when they are standing up than do women. Women have higher levels of a protein (heat-shock protein or Hsp 27) that protects and possibly repairs the esophageal lining from the more serious consequences of GERD—the constant assault of acid that can erode the lining of the esophagus, scar and narrow it, and even cause cancer. Pregnant women are at increased risk for GERD, possibly because of the impact of their high progesterone levels on esophageal contractions, which are longer and weaker during pregnancy. (When transsexual men received estrogen, they did not develop GERD, but when doctors added progesterone to their regimen, they often did.)

The Stomach

In the normal digestive process, food leaves a man's stomach a third faster than a woman's and liquids twice as quickly. Researchers don't know why this is true, but some believe that ovarian hormones, particularly progesterone, slow the process in women. As a result, women are more likely than men to feel overly full after eating and to experience troublesome belching after a meal. Many women have problems with abdominal bloating and gas immediately following a meal because of this slowdown in gut activity.

Pregnancy, with its riot of hormonal activity, can wreak havoc on a woman's digestive process. Most women experience nausea as soon as three weeks after a missed period, due to a disturbed gut "rhythm" that throws off sync the amplitude, frequency, and direction of the contractions that propel food forward (not unlike a cardiac arrhythmia, in which the regular beating of the heart is destabilized). The intensity of nausea during pregnancy is related to higher levels of progesterone and another hormone, human chorionic gonadotropin, as well as to *lower levels* of a hormone called motilin that modulates gut motility (movement of food through the system) during the nonpregnant state. These hormonal variations also contribute to the abdominal bloating and constipation that are so common during pregnancy. (This insight is a vast improvement over the attitude in the 1940s, when psychiatrists suggested that such symptoms were an attempt by the mother to reject the developing fetus, and postulated that such women were more likely to have had negative relationships with their own mothers.)

Sex-dependent differences in the lining of the stomach affect the incidence of certain diseases in men and women. For example, men secrete more stomach acid than women, possibly because testosterone stimulates the parietal (acid-producing) cells of the stomach. Estrogen is known to suppress acid secretion, and progesterone may have an added protective effect on the gastric lining. This difference may help to explain the fact that in a recent study of 1,456 patients, men were significantly more likely than women to develop duodenal ulcers (which are more likely to occur with higher exposure to stomach acid) when using nonsteroidal anti-inflammatory drugs (NSAIDs).[1]

The effects of hormones on the stomach lining can also help explain gender-specific differences in stomach cancers. In both men and women, for example, some cancers have receptors for estrogen and progesterone, and for patients whose cancers carry such receptors, survival rates are lower because circulating hormones attach to these receptors and impact the malignancy's behavior. The data are compelling enough that scientists have begun a trial of tamoxifen in patients with a specific kind of gastric cancer to see if it improves survival. (Tamoxifen is an estrogen-like molecule that attaches to the cancer's estrogen receptor, thus preventing estrogen from enhancing the tumor's growth.) Women with stomach cancer have higher-than-normal levels of serum progesterone; men with lower serum progesterone levels lived longer than other patients with the disease. Men whose cancers have been specifically tested for testosterone show lower-than-normal levels of the hormone. In fact, after surgery, testosterone levels in the blood of these men rose. It appears that the cancers themselves may regulate circulating hormone production, perhaps in a way that might optimize their own growth.

The Gallbladder

The liver manufactures a substance called bile (which is important for the proper digestion of fat) and stores it in a small, saclike organ called the gallbladder. The composition of bile is different in men and women. Estrogen and progesterone both increase the amount of cholesterol in bile. Progesterone also inhibits gallbladder contractions and therefore the frequency with which it empties its bile into the duodenum. Accordingly, gallbladder emptying is slower at the time of ovulation and during pregnancy, when progesterone levels are high. As a consequence, women develop gallbladder disease more frequently than men, particularly when they are carrying a child. For this reason, doctors recommend that patients who have gallstones have surgery before undertaking a pregnancy. Even after menopause, women are twice as likely as men to form gallstones; before menopause they have four times the risk!

The composition of bile varies both with the phases of the menstrual cycle and with pregnancy. Some of the breakdown products of bile in women increase their risk for colon cancer and may also explain the twice-higher incidence of inflammatory diseases of the intestine in females, such as ulcerative colitis and regional enteritis or Crohn's disease (an inflammation of the whole intestinal wall that can occur anywhere from the mouth to the anus but that is usually localized to the terminal ileum, the third part of the small intestine and the first part of the colon).

The Pancreas

If the vagaries of hormonal action on the gallbladder make women more vulnerable to gallbladder disease, the situation is reversed in the pancreas, where estrogen and progesterone seem to protect women from cancer. (Supporting this notion are studies showing that women who have had their ovaries removed before age fifty-five have a higher risk of developing pancreatic cancer.) Pancreatic cancer occurs three times more frequently in men than in women. Levels twice as high as normal of an enzyme (5-alpha reductase) that converts testosterone into its more potent form (5-alpha dihydrotestosterone) have been identified in patients with pancreatic cancer. These findings have been striking enough to make trials of treating pancreatic cancer with hormones seem reasonable.

The Intestine

THE ENTERIC NERVOUS SYSTEM

One of the most interesting and exciting discoveries about the intestine is that it has a complex and independent nervous system of its own, the *enteric nervous system* (ENS), which "thinks" for the gut and essentially governs how it functions. This "second brain," as Michael Gershon, professor of anatomy and cell biology at Columbia University's College of Physicians and Surgeons, calls it, has an intricate, two-way communication system with the brain; it explains why emotional stress causes such dramatic changes in bowel function. (Who among us has not had a feeling of nausea or an attack of diarrhea upon hearing very bad news or in response to severe stress?) Messages travel from the brain to the gut and back again over a special highway called the *vagus nerve.* Through this messaging circuit, the brain becomes aware of discomfort generated in the gut, and the gut responds to messages from the central nervous system. As Gershon puts it, "Whatever the exact connection, the relationship between the cerebral and enteric brains is so close that it is easy to become confused about which is doing the talking."[3]

But the ENS can function without the brain: the wave of muscular contractions that propels food along the intestinal tract (peristalsis) proceeds independently of any outside nervous input and is present even in a segment of gut that has been isolated from the body in the laboratory. In fact, the ENS acts like a pacemaker in the intestine, very much like the system of specialized, nervelike cells in the heart that initiates the cardiac beat and transmits it in an orderly fashion throughout the entire organ so that it contracts in a rhythmic, coordinated manner.

Like the neurons of the brain, the neurons of the ENS use many different chemicals (at least thirty, serotonin among them) to communicate with one another. The ENS's similarity to the brain doesn't end there: even the cells that form the support system encasing the axons of working nerve cells resemble those in the brain (astrocytes) that do the same thing for central nervous system neurons. Even more striking is the observation that lesions of the brain found in Parkinson's disease (Lewy bodies) and Alzheimer's disease (neurofibrillary tangles) are also to be found in the ENS. Gershon suggests that in the future we may be able to diagnose Alzheimer's disease by rectal biopsy!

One of Gershon's most provocative ideas is that when we use a selective serotonin-reuptake inhibitor to improve mood through its action on the central nervous system, we also inhibit serotonin uptake in the ENS. This explains why psychotropic drugs are so often accompanied by changes in bowel function. Almost a quarter of patients who begin to use an SSRI say they are nauseated or report diarrhea. Eventually, as doses are raised to produce the desired effect, the gut becomes desensitized to serotonin and patients develop constipation! Because of this "double action" of SSRIs, doctors are now using these medications to treat irritable bowel syndrome. Happily, gut function is normalized with far lower doses than are needed to improve mood, and IBS patients don't have the troublesome complication of constipation that higher doses produce.

IRRITABLE BOWEL SYNDROME

What is IBS, and how is it diagnosed? It is any of several disturbances of the intestine that cause pain, abdominal distention, and changes in the frequency and kind of stool eliminated. IBS is the most common of gastrointestinal disorders, affecting almost 15 percent of adults in Europe and China: 40 to 60 percent of people seen in gastrointestinal clinics have some form of this disorder. It affects three to six times more women than men. The cost and effort of treating this troublesome ailment in the United States is far from trivial, estimated at two million prescriptions and three million physician visits each year.

Before scientists developed their new understanding of how the gut works, and particularly the enteric nervous system, IBS was thought to be "all in the mind," the result of a neurotic personality. IBS is characterized by abdominal pain that is relieved by passing stool; more frequent bowel movements when pain begins; alterations in the frequency and consistency of stool; and abdominal distention. While doctors once concentrated almost exclusively on the colon in trying to diagnose and treat IBS, the pain is actually much more closely connected to malfunction of the small intestine. Food normally passes through this part of the gastrointestinal tract in an orderly three-phase process: a period of quiet (phase I) followed by a crescendo of random contractions (phase II) that finally culminate in effective, continuous phasic contractions (phase III). The patient with IBS never gets past phase II. This prolonged period of ineffective contractions is what seems to produce pain in the IBS sufferer. Women seem to sense this pain more intensely than do men. Just as doctors can map the rhythmic beating of the heart, they can also map the sequence of electrical impulses that "pace" the gut, moving food along with a coordinated series of contractions; in IBS, this regular pacing of the gut is disturbed and intense, resulting in ineffective and prolonged spasms of the intestine.

As scientists' understanding of the complex pattern of nervous activity that controls intestinal function deepened, it became obvious that, far from being a "psychological illness" lacking any real physical basis, IBS may well be the result of a disorder in the ENS, or a problem with central nervous system–ENS communication, or both. In addition to the complex nervous system that regulates the movement of food through the digestive tract, as scientists now know, other important factors also moderate gut motility, such as food intolerances and stress.

Certainly the *perception* of pain by patients with IBS differs from that of normal people: if the rectum is dilated with a balloon, IBS patients have spasms at lower levels of distention and report pain earlier than do nonaffected subjects. Women have a lower threshold than men for gut pain and experience more distress from it just before their menstrual periods. Females with IBS often have severe menstrual cramps as well. Women with IBS have a different pattern of blood flow in the brain than affected men, which may contribute to a more intense subjective experience of pain in females.

FUNCTIONAL BOWEL DISEASE

For women who don't meet the relatively rigid criteria for IBS, doctors have coined another term, *functional bowel disease* (FBD), essentially a catch-all term for gastrointestinal symptoms that can't be explained. Such symptoms—which include GERD, heartburn, nausea, vomiting, bloating, abdominal pain, and early fullness after eating—are often associated with another puzzling illness, fibromyalgia (a disorder characterized by muscle and joint pain, difficulty in sleeping and concentrating, and excessive fatigue; see Chapter 9). FBD is twenty times more common in women than in men, and its symptoms, like those of its sister disorder, IBS, fluctuate widely with hormonal changes: women often have worse symptoms premenstrually. Patients who are put on oral contraceptives that contain both estrogen and progestin often experience worsened FBS symptoms, while in postmenopausal women estrogen replacement *alone* had no impact on pain or distention, implying that progesterone is involved in causing the problem. A medication called alosetron that inhibits serotonin secretion is quite effective in women (but not men) who had diarrhea-predominant IBS and FBD; it has just been withdrawn from the market. The action of serotonin on the gut may be importantly impacted by gonadal hormones, which may be why women sufferers predominate in this disorder.

Very likely both IBS and FBD are overdiagnosed: 50 to 80 percent of problems referred to gastroenterologists are said to show "no pathology."[4] Patients (overwhelmingly women) and the physicians who are asked to evaluate their symptoms should be aware that specialized testing methods are now available that record the activity of the intestine over a period of several hours (very much as an electrocardiogram documents the rhythm of the heart) and hence can reveal a great deal about the cause of a patient's problems. The symptoms may be a result of malfunctioning nerves, those that supply the gut or those in the muscle of the intestinal wall itself. Nerve abnormalities are common in diseases like amyloidosis and diabetes, while smooth muscle disorders are a complication of scleroderma (a disease in which excessive amounts of collagen and other components of connective tissue are deposited in the skin and internal organs; 50 percent of scleroderma patients have gastrointestinal involvement).

Myoelectric disorders, which include IBS, are the result of faulty pacing of the gut's activity. A particularly interesting myoelectric disorder is tachygastria (seen almost exclusively in young women) in which an abnormal "pacesetter" in the terminal part of the stomach fires six to eight times a minute and causes food to be pushed in the wrong direction, delaying gastric emptying. Patients feel full after only a few mouthfuls of food and feel nauseated and vomit soon after eating. Some young women have required removal of the distal stomach for a cure.

Sometimes what is misdiagnosed as IBS is actually due to bacterial toxins circulating in the blood or within the gut itself, acting like laxatives.

Finally, hormonal fluxes, or increased sensitivity to the action of hormones, are a common cause of problems, particularly in women, many of whom experience diarrhea on the first day of their menstrual cycles.

COLON CANCER: WHY COLONOSCOPY AFTER FIFTY IS IMPERATIVE

Many women have an almost pathological fear of breast cancer but worry much less about the third most common malignancy in women, colon cancer. Despite the far-graver consequences of colon cancer, they resist having a colonoscopy (an internal exam). As my favorite gastroenterologist once commented, "Is it better to have a colonoscopy now, or intra-arterial chemotherapy for a cancer we find too late?" Unfortunately, colon cancer is usually asymptomatic until it is quite advanced. The disease is even worse for women; a typical colon cancer in women is located 10 to 20 percent higher up in the colon than in men, and a sigmoidoscopy (which doesn't go far enough to examine the whole colon) is no guarantee that there isn't a cancer growing beyond the reach of the examining scope.

In six out of seven studies, cholecystectomy (removal of the gallbladder) was found to increase the risk for colon cancer, so women who have had their gallbladders removed should be monitored more carefully than others. Removing the gallbladder results in a *continuous* secretion of bile into the intestine, whereas when bile stays stationary for a time in the gallbladder, its composition changes, and it may be less irritating to the colon as a result. Women who use HRT have 33 percent less risk for colon cancer than same-age women not on HRT.

Relatively young women (less than fifty-five) seem to be at higher risk than older women, implying that estrogen and/or progesterone may influence susceptibility to colon cancer.

METABOLISM, WEIGHT, AND EATING DISORDERS

Gender and Obesity

We are definitely living in the age of the cult of youth; woman after woman comes into my office asking about cosmetic surgery—and they're doing so at younger and younger ages. But in spite of all the warnings about overweight and all our national efforts to control, reduce, or eliminate obesity (officially defined as a body mass index—weight in kilograms divided by height in centimeters—of 30 or higher), Americans are fatter than ever. Thirty-four percent of American women and 31.2 percent of men are overweight. Among women, there are important racial differences: black (48.6 percent) and Mexican American (47.2 percent) women are generally heavier than Caucasian women (33.2 percent). The data for overweight men are strikingly different: white and black men have nearly identical numbers (31.6 percent and 31.2 percent), while 39.2 percent of Mexican American men are overweight. According to a survey done by the Commonwealth Fund's Commission on Women's Health, women had an additional problem: their *perception* of whether they were fat or thin often did not correspond to reality. Forty-three percent of women who were actually of normal size thought they were overweight. Four out of ten women under sixty-five and one out of four over sixty-five were trying to lose weight: 60 percent were consuming fewer calories and 40 percent were also actively exercising. Interestingly, only 6 percent were using weight loss programs.

Metabolism: The Balance of Calories and Energy

Think about this: over an entire lifetime, each of us ingests a total of *50 million calories* (which amounts to eighteen tons of food or six tons of pure fat). Obviously, we don't gain anywhere near that much weight—most of us put on an average of only *thirty-three pounds* over the course of our entire adult life.[5] How, then, does the body balance the food we take in with the calories we burn to stay alive and move around the planet?

Metabolism is a complex issue, one scientists don't fully understand. Any model we come up with must account for exceptions, like the chubby woman who sits across from me weeping as she explains that she eats fewer than 800 calories a day, exercises, and still can't lose weight. Such women have usually been heavy all their lives and are sometimes the only overweight member of their families. In the past, doctors were convinced that these women were either unconsciously or consciously deceiving themselves, and everyone else, about what they actually ate during the day. Other women, often the daughters of women who were obsessed with weight and were constantly dieting, arrive in my office, sent there by other physicians or even by their mothers who gave them diet pills when they were thirteen years old and insisted they fast for weight control. Some of these patients look skeletally thin, and others seem quite healthy and of normal weight, but they are plagued by anorexia (an obsessive refusal to eat enough calories to maintain weight), bulimia (vomiting just ingested food to prevent it from being metabolized and converted to tissue), or binge eating. In these women, something has happened to disturb the remarkable system of checks and balances that the body uses to keep our size constant, enabling us to sense quite accurately how big we are and how much food we need to eat to keep our body mass constant.

The Story of Leptin

In 1998 scientists discovered a remarkable new hormone, produced in fat cells themselves, that signals the brain that the body has had enough to eat and quenches appetite for more food. Called *leptin* (from the Greek word *leptos,* meaning "thin"), it is also called the satiety hormone, and its discovery sparked new hope for weight control.

Leptin was studied first in mice. Researchers found that mice that could not produce leptin (because of a genetic defect) ate constantly and became grossly overweight; they had no sense of when they had eaten enough food to satisfy themselves. Giving them leptin immediately restored their ability to become satiated, and they quickly returned to normal weight. Leptin acts on the part of the brain called the hypothalamus, one of the most important centers for appetite control. Here a "hunger hormone" called *neuropeptidase Y* is produced, which drives animals (and people) to eat. Researchers found receptors for leptin on the surface of the very same cells that produce neuropeptidase Y; when leptin reaches the brain, it locks onto these cells, "turning off" the production of neuropeptidase Y, and turning off appetite with it.

Imagine doctors' excitement when they learned of these astonishing experiments. But the story, unfortunately, is not as simple for humans as it is for mice. In the first place, mutations in the gene that controls leptin production are exceedingly rare in humans, so blaming obesity on a genetic flaw in ourselves is more difficult than in rodents! In the second place, although leptin levels were undetectable in the mice with the genetic defect, leptin levels were very high in obese humans, particularly in women. So what is the problem? Why, if we have normal or even very high levels of leptin, do we continue to gain weight and, presumably, eat more than we need? The answer might be one of three possibilities. First, we might have *defective receptors* for leptin: in spite of an abundance of hormone, leptin can't attach to the abnormal receptor and "turn off" the cells producing the hunger hormone, neuropeptidase Y. Another possibility is that in spite of plenty of leptin in the blood, it cannot cross from the cerebrospinal fluid that bathes the brain into the brain itself. It might be blocked by what scientists call a *transport defect*. Other researchers find no evidence that this is the case and believe in a third possibility—that some primary defect in the brain itself makes it unresponsive to leptin. In this crucial sense, we are very different from mice: we have plenty of leptin, especially if we are female, but some barrier is preventing its effective use.

In general, women's leptin levels are almost twice those of men. Once their body fat rises above 25 percent of their total body weight, women's leptin levels rise three times higher than those of men as they put on extra pounds. Hormones do not explain women's higher leptin levels; even after menopause, women continue to have higher levels than men, levels that are no different from those of younger women.

Some experts think that women may have a resistance or lower sensitivity to leptin than men, which would explain why females have more body fat than males and why women find it harder to maintain their newly reduced weight after dieting than do men. Difficulty maintaining a lower weight may also be related to the fact that leptin levels remain low for at least two months after weight loss, in spite of a return to an unrestricted diet.

Leptin secretion varies during a twenty-four-hour period; it is highest at night, perhaps to inhibit hunger during sleep. In mice, at least, it is lowest at about four P.M.; some patients describe excessive fatigue (relieved only by food) at that time of day. These rhythmic changes in leptin concentration disappear if we fast, which makes levels rise and stay elevated both day and night. This may explain some of the loss of interest in food that prolonged fasting produces.

Among scientists, interest in leptin continues to increase. Currently more than six hundred scientific papers have been published on the subject. All agree that it has an important role in satiety, signaling when an animal or person has had enough to eat. But it has other important functions too. Although leptin is generally produced by fat cells in the subcutaneous tissue just under the skin, it has also been found in the placenta (where it may serve as an important signal for energy status between mother and fetus), liver, muscle, pancreas, and intestine. In the fetus, it is produced by an even wider range of tissues. Leptin is also an important fertility hormone; it can restore the ability of an animal to ovulate and is probably important as the signal for menses to begin in the adolescent girl, and for ejaculation in the adolescent male. It also prevents the loss of ovulation and the declining levels of testosterone that occur with starvation in humans. Overall, leptin turns out to have a much more complicated role in the body's upkeep than we expected; though it may not prove to be the Holy Grail of weight loss, an improved understanding of its function can only help us in our quest to understand the human body and how its functions differ in men and women.

Gender and Body Fat

If leptin regulates overall body mass, what factors are responsible for women's and men's different body shapes? Classically, women look like pears and men like apples. Women carry more fat "on" their bodies and deposit most of it in three areas: breasts, hips, and buttocks. Men, on the other hand, carry their fat "within" the body; they tend to accumulate it in the abdominal area and around the intestines. Androgens (the male hormones, one of which is testosterone) also make men's muscle mass higher and their bones heavier than women's.

This sex-specific distribution of body fat is determined importantly by our hormones: the more androgynous a person is, the more he or she is inclined to deposit fat around the midsection. Women with polycystic ovary syndrome (an endocrine problem characterized by infertility, obesity, and a male distribution of body hair) have higher levels of androgens than average women and significantly higher waist-hip ratios (the circumference of the waist divided by the circumference of the hips). Some aspect of hormone balance is genetic. Of all women measured in the European Fat Distribution Study, Mediterranean women had the highest free testosterone concentrations and the greatest abdominal girth.

As any woman who has borne a child can tell you, body shape changes significantly with reproduction. The cause is changes in the activity of an enzyme involved in the metabolism of fat (lipoprotein lipase) and in the sensitivity of fat cells to insulin. Body fat is redistributed during pregnancy, when the amount of fat in the upper legs decreases. After reaching a peak in the second trimester, body fat begins to decrease in the third. If the new baby is nursed, the mother accumulates fat in the breasts, upper arms, and upper trunk. By about six months after lactation, her body fat distribution returns to baseline levels.

Eating Disorders

Eating disorders are just that: profound distortions in how we take in food. Contrary to popular opinion, both sexes are affected by these problems, though the illnesses manifest themselves differently and are most effectively treated in different ways.

Perhaps the best-known eating disorder is *anorexia nervosa,* in which the patient has a distorted sense of how large his or her body actually is. Patients feel fat, even when they are painfully thin. They have a preoccupation with body shape too and often exercise compulsively to keep their weight at a minimum and to "define" muscle groups and "perfect" the contours of their body. Food intake is kept to a minimum, even to the point of literal starvation. In fact, the death rate associated with anorexia is twelve times higher than that of the same-age population; 0.56 percent of anorexics die each year.

Bulimia is a disorder characterized by binge eating, when the patient loses control over how much food he or she eats at a single sitting. Then, alarmed at the possibility of weight gain after an episode of overeating, the patient takes extreme measures to avoid weight gain, including the use of diuretics or laxatives and self-induced vomiting. Even these measures don't completely neutralize the effect of all that food, so unlike anorexics, bulimics often have a completely normal body size. In fact, in a recent Scandinavian study,[6] body mass index was significantly higher in adolescent bulimics than in healthy children. Doctors have learned to look for telltale signs, though, like scratches on the back of the hand from inducing vomiting and damage to tooth enamel from stomach acid, as well as more subtle signs like electrocardiographic abnormalities and low pulse rate.

Menstrual periods can stop in any kind of eating disorder, but they stop more commonly in patients with anorexia, who severely restrict their food intake. In these women, leptin levels are low and reproductive function ceases; the signals the brain sends via the pituitary gland (through gonadotropin-releasing hormone, produced in the hypothalamus) to the ovaries and testes fail. Although doctors tend to look more carefully at females for evidence of bulimic behavior, a full 40 percent of bulimics are boys and men. As research progresses, scientists are finding that eating disorders are actually common in boys involved in sports that require low body weight like gymnastics. Males also may experience an eating disorder called *reverse anorexia* or *bulking* in which competitive athletes use steroids and high caloric intake to build large muscles quickly.

What causes an eating disorder? Societal standards of what is beautiful clearly have an important impact on what people believe about body size, but the causes are complicated and manifold: genes, parental example, brain chemistry, and even socioeconomic status all contribute to the development of anorexia and bulimia.

Unlike other psychiatric illnesses, eating disorders are culturally specific: in societies where food is scarce, they don't exist. They occur only in situations where thinness is equated with beauty, and where there is a surplus of available food. The media certainly play a part. In a fascinating study about the impact of television on body image, Harvard anthropologist Anne Becker studied what happened in the Fiji Islands to young girls exposed to TV images from the United States, Britain, and Australia. Fiji culture traditionally emphasizes the importance of food: guests are expected to eat as much as possible, often well beyond the point at which they feel satisfied. Eighty-four percent of Fiji women were classified as overweight or obese, and their diets were very high in fat. The culture approved of this large body size; in fact, when a Fiji islander began to lose weight, it was assumed that some problem had caused the person to "go thin," and he or she was given herbal remedies to restore appetite.

This situation changed entirely when TV came to the island in 1995. Within three years the number of young girls who admitted vomiting to control their weight had increased fivefold! Those who watched TV more than three nights a week were 50 percent more likely to see themselves as too fat and 30 percent more likely to diet. This was true in spite of the fact that frequent and infrequent TV watchers had no difference in body size.

In addition to popular notions of beauty and fitness, other factors affect body image as well. Eating disorders are more frequent, for example, in groups that value slender bodies (like ballet dancers) and in families in which dieting is inappropriately and prematurely emphasized. One patient told me of modeling her new Easter dress for her father when she was only ten years old. Her father said, "I hope you're not going to be one of those soft little fatties you go to school with!" My patient never forgot the remark and never felt the same about her body. Her lifelong preoccupation with being thin, I believe, had its roots in that moment. In treating her I explained that preadolescent girls characteristically have very little waistline definition, and that their relatively increased abdominal girth is part of the necessary mass of body fat that has to be achieved before menses can begin.

One of the most important new discoveries about eating disorders is that they don't occur only in late adolescence. Careful studies show that they increasingly occur in young children and can even begin after forty years of age. Males are affected too; they're not just diseases of females. Doctors underdiagnose eating disorders in boys and men, partially because they don't believe males are susceptible and partly because they are not familiar with the different ways men and women experience eating disorders.

Men feel thin at weights up to 105 percent of normal; women, on the other hand, consider themselves thin when they are at only 87 percent of their ideal weight. Men are most likely to be dissatisfied with their upper bodies, while women are usually discontented with what is below their waists. Women diet because they believe being thin is its own reward, while men diet for any of several reasons: in response to childhood teasing about being fat; to improve their athletic prowess (particularly in wrestling or gymnastics); to avoid the medical illnesses associated with obesity; or because of a homosexual relationship. (Twenty percent of men with eating disorders are homosexual,[7] and the incidence of eating disorders in male homosexuals is four times that of eating disorders in the general population.) One type of eating disorder, reverse anorexia, occurs almost entirely in males but sometimes appears in females involved in sports like competitive swimming, who are interested in bulking up their bodies and have a pathological fear of being not too fat, but too thin!

Some of the consequences of anorexia are common to both genders: young adult female anorexics often have the bone density of eighty-year-old women,[8] and data suggest that the problem in anorexic males is just as profound. Even more interestingly, although testosterone levels and the amount of weight loss correlate with bone density, neither men nor women show an improvement in bone density with testosterone or estrogen therapy *as long as body weight remains low.*

Treatment of eating disorders should therefore differ according to the sex of the patient. If a male anorexic is simply encouraged to gain weight in a hospital treatment unit, then leaves with a thickened waistline, he will relapse. It's particularly important, therefore, for anorexic men to combine increased caloric intake with physical activity and the counseling of a trainer, so that their upper body shape remains optimal. Sexual counseling is important too, and again it should differ, depending on the sex of the patient: women anorexics are most commonly either asexual or sexually timid, while sexual identity conflicts and problems are almost entirely specific to males. In contrast to men, sexual abuse is a frequent antecedent of anorexia in women, so this possibility should be carefully explored in therapy, which is more successful in females if it is one on one. Group therapy for men seems to be more effective if it is restricted to all male patients; the treatment teams for men should include male professionals, although once a therapeutic bond is established, the sex of the therapist doesn't seem to be important to a successful outcome.

WHAT DOES THE NEW SCIENCE MEAN FOR YOU?

Is there anything special that women need to know or do to take care of their mouth and teeth?

- At puberty, gum infection (gingivitis) is three times more common in girls than in boys.
- During menstruation, increased susceptibility to gum infection can develop into a stubborn case of serious gingivitis, so paying scrupulous attention to flossing and brushing is even more important during your menstrual period than during the rest of the month.
- During pregnancy, infection and bleeding of the gums are common problems. Pockets of infected, exuberantly growing gum tissue can actually look like tumors, particularly in the second and eighth months of pregnancy. During this vulnerable time, be prepared to see your dentist more often, at least in the first and last trimesters.

- Menopausal women often experience a dry or burning mouth, as well as loosened teeth, as a result of osteoporosis. Zinc deficiency is not uncommon in older patients; it results in an altered, even dulled sense of taste.
- If you have an eating disorder like bulimia, in addition to considering counseling and treatment for the disorder, you may want to see a dentist, as acid from your stomach may have eroded your tooth enamel and damaged soft tissue in the mouth.
- Tongue piercing with rings or buttons can result in difficulty with speech and produce infections that are difficult to treat while the decoration remains in place. These infections also cause particularly bad breath because of the kind of bacteria that collect in the mouth. Traction on the ring can also cause serious tongue laceration.

What are the signs of GERD?

Often the only symptom of GERD is a persistent and disturbing cough that makes even sleep impossible. Awakening from sleep choking is another signal that you need attention. If you have a cough without a fever, a cold, or any other symptoms, ask your doctor if GERD is a possibility. She will probably suggest you try a medicine like omeprazole (Prilosec) or famotidine (Pepcid) to inhibit acid production in your stomach.

How do I know that the severe pain I experience in my chest isn't a heart attack?

Severe, intermittent pain in the center of the chest that's due to esophageal spasm can exactly mimic the pain of a heart attack. It should be called to the attention of a doctor *immediately*. After ruling out coronary artery disease (with a stress echocardiogram, if you are a woman), your doctor may recommend a test that monitors the concentration of esophageal acidity over a twenty-four-hour period. She may also send you for direct measurements of the strength of your esophageal contractions, to decide whether the problem is cardiac or gastrointestinal. Then she will plan a course of treatment.

I've complained for years about abdominal pain and diarrhea alternating with constipation, but doctors haven't found the cause. Am I just a hypochondriac?

Admittedly, doctors know very little about functional bowel disorder and irritable bowel syndrome and still have difficulty treating their symptoms. But even if you are diagnosed with FBD instead of IBS, ask for a trial on one of the SSRI medications like fluoxetine (Prozac) or paroxetine (Paxil). You might have a real improvement in symptoms.

I have tremendous problems with belching, abdominal distention, and flatulence every time I eat anything. What causes it, and what can I do about it?

Any change in your digestive function that lasts over a week is worth a visit to your doctor. The problem can be due to a number of factors, but your doctor can help you decide what the best first steps are. To begin with, tell your doctor about any recent travel, even if it's within the United States. Parasitic infestation is not unusual after a camping trip to some areas, and travel overseas may produce infection, which usually appears as acute stomach pain and diarrhea a few hours after eating. These types of parasitic infections are simply detected and easily treated. Two weeks after you complete the course of medicine your doctor has ordered, you should be retested to see if the infestation is over.

If the problem is chronic, discuss simple changes in your dietary habits with your doctor. For example,

- Eat smaller and more frequent meals, rather than large meals consumed at a single sitting, to give your gut more time to process the food. This is a particularly good idea during pregnancy, when esophageal reflux and increased transit time for food are common problems.
- Add small amounts of *soluble* fiber to your diet. Foods rich in soluble fiber include oatmeal, pasta, rice, French bread, and sourdough bread. *Insoluble* fiber (whole wheat bran, raw fruit and vegetables, and sprouts) *may only make the problem worse* by stimulating the gastrointestinal tract and increasing its water content.

- Keep a food diary for a month so that you can note any connection between specific foods and an increase in symptoms. The most common troublesome foods are dairy products, cabbage, beans, apples, grape juice, bananas, nuts, and raisins.
- Avoid caffeine, nicotine, chocolate, alcohol, spicy foods, and large, high-fat meals; all are common offenders, even for completely normal guts!

Before your doctor labels a persistent series of complaints "functional," she should do appropriate testing to rule out treatable illnesses and even in some cases to avoid surgery. To rule out localized or generalized motility disturbances in the gut, several tests are available. These include tracing the progress of radioactive labeled food or pellets through the gastrointestinal tract and measuring the gut's activity directly with a probe. Definable disorders (such as gastrointestinal motor dysfunction, pseudo-obstruction syndromes, hollow visceral neuropathy, and myopathy) can be diagnosed with careful testing and are no longer called "functional" bowel disorders.

My doctor wanted to do a rectal examination as part of my annual checkup, but I refused. Why did he suggest this?

Most primary care physicians don't do a rectal examination on women, but it can be a vitally important part of their preventive care, particularly for those over fifty and for those who have had their gallbladders removed. *An annual test of your stool for occult blood* (small amounts of blood that may not be apparent to the patient) *is as important as a mammogram or a Pap smear.* A positive test may signal the presence of a colonic polyp that will inevitably become malignant.

I've been fighting anorexia for ten years. How can I find out if I've done permanent damage to myself?

People with eating disorders are not all skeletally thin, not all obviously emotionally disturbed, and *not all female.* They can appear quite normal but may have done significant damage to their bodies. Some of the issues include

- Erosion of tooth enamel
- Pancreatic disease due to repeated bouts of overeating, particularly foods laden with fats
- Dangerous thinning of the skeleton with osteoporosis and fractures even in late adolescence
- Infertility and loss of menstrual periods

If you have had an eating disorder in the past but are now eating normally again, you may still need a bone density test to check whether you have enough bone strength for protection against fractures. Extra rations of calcium and even bisphosphonates, which rebuild bone, might be indicated.

If you have an eating disorder severe enough to have lost your menstrual period, you should talk to your doctor about oral contraceptives to protect your bones.

A selective serotonin-reuptake inhibitor might help if you are bulimic. And in all cases of eating disorders, if you aren't currently being treated, you should explore avenues of counseling and support. Ask your doctor to recommend a therapist or support group. Countless programs and therapists are devoted entirely to addressing these kinds of disorders. You do not have to endure these issues alone.

My son is a varsity gymnast and is scrupulous about keeping his weight low. He refuses to eat meals with others in restaurants or even at home with the family. He seems quite healthy and, of course, exercises all the time. Should I be worried?

Your son may very well have an eating disorder. They aren't restricted to adolescent girls but are quite common in male athletes engaged in sports for which low body weight is a requirement, and in male dancers. It's important to talk to your son *as well as his coaches and teachers* about this problem so he doesn't compromise his bone mass and eats the amount and variety of foods he needs to support normal growth and adequate nutrition. By the way, if he is bulimic (vomiting after eating) or purging (using laxatives to expel food), both practices are usually kept secret from family and friends, which may be why he's so reclusive at mealtimes. If he complains from time to time about excessive fatigue, this could be the consequence of low potassium levels in his blood from laxative use. Taken to extremes, potassium deficiency can produce dangerous disturbances in the heart's rhythm and can even cause fatal cardiac arrest. Eating disorders are not just a personal choice, to be ignored or minimized; they can be fatal.

CHAPTER 5

The Heart and Circulatory System

IN 1987 A group of courageous investigators made a remarkable and disturbing discovery that began a revolution in health care. Tobin and Steingart showed that cardiologists were treating the complaints of men and women very differently: doctors were twice as likely to ascribe a woman's symptoms to hysteria or emotion as those of a man![1] Astonishingly, this pattern turned out to be true even when actors—one male and the other female—read *an identical script describing cardiac symptoms to the doctor.* Worse still, women whose exercise-thallium tests (a test that traces the distribution of blood through the coronary arteries at the peak of exercise) produced abnormal results were *ten times less likely* to be referred for cardiac catheterization, the definitive test for coronary artery disease (CAD).* Subsequent studies have documented even more troubling news: women were receiving much more conservative *treatment* for their CAD than were men. While doctors prescribed medicines for women, they were sending men for aggressive

---

* In this test, the cardiologist threads a catheter into the heart through an artery in the leg, pushing it past the valve that separates the left ventricle from the great artery that carries fresh, oxygenated blood to the body, the aorta. She then injects dye through the catheter into the right and the left coronary arteries, the first branches of the aorta that carry blood to the heart muscle itself. The resulting picture of the coronary arteries tells doctors whether there is obstruction, and where it is located in the heart.

interventions like clot-buster therapy, angioplasty, or coronary artery bypass surgery.* Women's CAD was—and is still—more likely to be managed by medication than by more aggressive intervention. Whether this is because doctors make more conservative decisions for female patients than they do for males or because women themselves choose more conservative therapy is still unclear. It is possible, some experts say, that women are having just the right treatment and that men are being treated too aggressively.

Whatever the case may be, women are less likely to receive recommended medications for management of the abnormal serum lipids (the fats carried in the bloodstream, like cholesterol and triglycerides) that are serious risk factors for heart disease. They are also less likely than men to receive medicines that have been proven to prolong life once a patient has had a heart attack.

Women were shocked by these findings. Happily, so were their physicians. Along with many of my colleagues, I was part of the revolution that resulted. The cardiovascular community of researching scientists and practicing physicians all rose to the challenge. Because of these findings more women were included in studies of heart disease. Until the 1990s, almost all the information we had about the cardiovascular system came from studies done exclusively on men—in spite of the fact that cardiovascular disease kills more women each year than all cancers combined! The new findings about men's and women's hearts have established one of the most important bodies of information in the new science of gender-specific medicine.

---

* Angioplasty is a procedure in which a catheter threaded into a blocked artery carries an expandable balloon or other device for destroying plaque in the artery. (Plaque is made of cholesterol, calcium, clot, and other elements.) Coronary artery bypass surgery (CABG) is a procedure in which part of a blood vessel is harvested from the body (a leg vein or an artery in the chest or wrist) and is grafted onto the diseased coronary artery above the point of obstruction. The other end is grafted below the obstructed area, so that blood is routed around the obstruction and bypasses it completely.

THE NORMAL HEART

The heart is a four-chambered muscular organ that receives blood from the veins of the body into its two right chambers. The lower right chamber, the right ventricle, pumps the blood to the lungs, where it is purified and resupplied with oxygen. The freshened blood then returns from the lungs via the pulmonary veins to the left side of the heart, the lower chamber of which, the left ventricle, then pumps it forward into the aorta and its branches, which distribute it throughout the body, where it purifies and nourishes our tissues and organs.

Like every part of the body, the size of the heart is proportional to the size of the whole person, so in general, women's hearts are smaller than those of men. But women do not necessarily have smaller coronary arteries than men. Still, doctors have justified not sending women with severe coronary artery disease on to open-heart surgery because they have been told that women's arteries are too small for bypass surgery. This is not the case; artery size in women varies widely, and most are entirely suitable for bypass. Women *have* had a higher mortality rate than men in bypass surgery, but this is because women were often diagnosed much later than men and were therefore older and sicker when they were referred for the operation. Now that doctors have learned to recognize the unique symptoms of CAD in women and how to test women more accurately, they diagnose them sooner. In centers where experienced surgeons perform bypass surgery on a daily basis, women now do as well as men in terms of survival.

Men, Women, and the Heartbeat

The heart beats because it generates its own electrical impulse in a special nodule of tissue, the sinus node, in the upper part of the right chamber called the atrium. This impulse travels throughout the entire heart along specialized conducting pathways, very much like electrical wiring, and stimulates the heart muscle to contract. An *electrocardiogram* (ECG) is a device that records the electrical activity of the heart, allowing the physician to see, among other things, whether the electrical impulse spreads through the heart muscle normally and whether each stage in the process is completed within a normal amount of time.

Each of the complexes that make up a heartbeat is composed of three different parts, and each part is named with a letter. Thus, a single cardiac impulse on the electrocardiogram has a P wave, a sequence of deflections called the QRS complex, and a T wave. The P wave represents the excitation of the upper chambers of the heart (the atria), the QRS complex that of the lower chambers (the ventricles), and the T wave the time it takes for the excited tissue to return to a resting state. The part of the ECG that indicates how long the heart takes to return to a resting state so that it can be excited by the next beat is called the Q-T interval. During the first part of that interval, the heart cannot be excited at all. During the last part of it, though, as it begins to return to a resting state, it is more excitable than usual and is susceptible to destabilization or capture by beats that arise in areas outside the normal electrical network of the heart. These are called *ectopic* beats and are almost always premature: they take control of the heart before the next normal beat has time to develop.

Normal women are more likely than men to develop early or premature beats and even prolonged periods of very rapid abnormal beating (called arrhythmias). Why? Doctors have known for decades, since ECGs were first invented, that certain features of the ECG are normally different in males and females as soon as children achieve puberty. At puberty, boys' Q-T intervals shorten under the influence of testosterone. This makes sexually mature men's hearts more resistant to extra beats than women's. The longer Q-T of women makes it more likely that an extra beat will capture the heart's rhythm and start an arrhythmia. This vulnerability of women is influenced by hormonal shifts, perhaps profoundly. Many women complain that their heart palpitations become worse just before or early in their menstrual cycles. In fact, in one study of women with arrhythmias, 59 percent of patients reported that these periods of abnormal rhythm were associated with hormonal shifts—and 41 percent felt that hormonal shifts were the only precipitating factor. Estrogen can make the heart susceptible to abnormal rhythms; it intensifies the sensitivity of the heart to input from the *sympathetic* nervous system. (The sympathetic nervous system is part of the *autonomic* nervous system that controls the functions of the body that are not consciously regulated; the rate at which I breathe, for example, and the rate at which my heart beats are not something I consciously regulate; it happens automatically. The *parasympathetic* nervous system—the other part of the autonomic nervous system—slows the heart rate, while the sympathetic nervous system speeds it up.) In fact, the first oral contraceptive pills on the market, which had much higher estrogen concentrations than the pills we now use, increased abnormal beats in women with no underlying heart disease. In men, exercise is more often a trigger for abnormal rhythms; in women, hormonal *fluxes* or changes in levels are more likely to cause them.

Perimenopausal women (women who are still having menstrual periods but are also experiencing periods of estrogen deficiency as their ovarian function slows down) complain of palpitations more than younger women. Many times they have never had them before. This phenomenon too is hormone-related; low doses of estrogen often eliminate such symptoms.

Ironically, some of the very drugs developed to control and eliminate arrhythmias create unique problems for women. Why? Because many of them work by prolonging the time the heart takes to relax after each beat. In women, in whom this process already takes a relatively longer time, such a drug creates a paradoxical situation in which the patient is more likely to develop extra beats that often crescendo into arrhythmia. One of these arrhythmic patterns, which is particularly dangerous, is called *torsades de pointes* (a French phrase that literally means "revolving around a horizontal line" because of its characteristic chaotic pattern on the electrocardiogram), a potentially fatal event. Pharmaceutical companies are now trying to develop anti-arrhythmic drugs for women that diminish the instability of their heartbeat rather than increase it. Women are more likely to suffer sudden cardiac death than men during anti-arrhythmic therapy, and in one study of drug trials carried out between 1980 and 1992, women made up 70 percent of drug-related torsades de pointes.

The Heart Muscle: What's Unique to Each Sex?

The bulk of the heart, which does the work of receiving and pumping blood to the body, is a unique kind of muscle. And just like the specialized cells that make up the electrical system of the heart, this tissue is different in men and women.

Cardiac muscle, like muscle everywhere in the body, is made up of individual units called *contractile proteins*. The composition of these proteins is different for males and females, which may explain why certain aspects of the efficiency with which the heart pumps blood differs between men and women. There are other differences too: individual muscle cells and groups of cells are held together in a mechanically well-integrated network by fiberlike, structural materials that form a kind of skeleton on which the muscle cells are arranged. Women have more of this supporting tissue than do men, which may account for the increasing stiffness of the heart in aging women, whose hearts are unable to work as efficiently as when they were younger: they have lost some of the important elasticity that lets the heart expand to receive blood between beats. Recent studies of congestive heart failure in women show that the cause might be increased stiffness or loss of elasticity of their heart muscle more than is the case for men, who are more likely to have a problem with weakened muscle fibers.

Some of these sex-specific differences in the composition of the heart are under the control of hormones. In animals, for example, thyroid hormone stimulates the growth of normal connective tissue (collagen) in the heart, and its effect is much more pronounced in males. Hypothyroidism (a disease in which the thyroid becomes less active than normal) is more common in women than in men. Women with hypothyroidism have much less elastic heart muscle than normal women.

CARDIOVASCULAR DISEASE: HOW DOES IT DIFFER FOR MEN AND WOMEN?

High Blood Pressure (Hypertension)

Blood pressure is literally the force exerted on the wall of a blood vessel by the blood contained within it. Because there is more blood in the arterial system when the heart contracts, the pressure is higher; when the heart relaxes, the amount of fluid in the vessels is less. When your doctor tells you your blood pressure is 140 over 80, she means that when your heart contracts (the systolic blood pressure), the pressure in your arteries is equal to that of the weight of 140 milliliters of mercury (mm Hg) and that when your heart relaxes (the diastolic blood pressure) it is equal to that of 80 mm Hg. Women, at least until menopause, have lower blood pressure while they are awake than men of the same ages and a bigger dip in blood pressure at night. This difference emerges at the time of puberty. By about sixty, however, high blood pressure is more often found in women than in men. The protection that younger women enjoy thus seems to be related to ovarian hormone secretion, a concept that is borne out by animal studies: castrating young male rats reduced their blood pressure, while removing the ovaries of female rats caused their pressure to rise.

Officially, any blood pressure measurement that is higher than 140/90 mm Hg is called high and the patient has *hypertension*. More recently, doctors have found that 130/80 mm Hg is a safer limit for women and one at which the tissues of the body are best perfused with blood at an acceptable level of work by the heart.

The response of the heart to a need for increased work is different as a function of gender. When men develop high blood pressure, the major pumping chamber of the heart (the left ventricle) increases the size of muscle cells and the amount of connective tissue supporting those cells, so that it can push blood forward even with higher-than-normal pressure in the arteries. When this happens in a man, his ventricle becomes bigger, but the thickness of the wall does not increase. Women, on the other hand, meet the challenge by developing thicker-walled left ventricles; there is much less change in the overall size of the chamber, but it has a smaller interior surrounded by a thicker rim of muscle. This is called *concentric left ventricular hypertrophy* (LVH). Both sexes, then, increase muscle mass to pump blood against higher pressure, but the geometry of the bigger (hypertrophied) heart is different for men and women. This means that hypertensive women's thicker-walled hearts may be less elastic than those of men's, which may be a disadvantage for females. LVH is associated with a 50 percent higher rate of cardiovascular disorders in women than in men, and hypertension or high blood pressure is associated with stroke in 59 percent of women but only 39 percent of men.

About a quarter of all the people in the world have high blood pressure, and about 60 percent of them are women. Doctors never discover the reason for most hypertension, so hypertension with unknown causes is called *essential hypertension*. But in a small percentage of cases, particularly in patients under the age of thirty-five in whom there is no family history of high blood pressure, the causes are known. For example, in young people, the artery to the kidney may become narrowed, whereupon the kidney, experiencing lower-than-normal blood flow, begins to manufacture a chemical, angiotensin, that is a potent constrictor of arteries and makes blood pressure go up. Angiotensin also causes retention of salt and water, increasing the amount of fluid within the intra-arterial compartment and pushing pressure up still further. Eight times as many females as males develop this condition; doctors are not sure why.

Oral contraceptives are another cause of hypertension in women. With the older pills, which had a higher dose of estrogen than the present ones, about 5 percent of the women who took them developed high blood pressure, which never returned to normal in about 50 percent of those women, even after they stopped the pill. Modern versions of oral contraceptives have a lower dose of estrogen, and the risk of developing high blood pressure is less, though it is still about double the risk of women not on the pill. Women who use the tricyclic formula, because it has the lowest levels of progesterone, are at the lowest risk of all women using oral contraceptives for developing hypertension.

The situation seems to be quite different for women using HRT after menopause; in fact, in the older patient, estrogen may help to prevent hypertension, particularly in the patch (rather than the oral form).

Although much more study is needed to determine conclusively whether men and women respond differently to the hypertension medicines currently available, evidence suggests that they do. For example, in women, the use of a thiazide diuretic (a class of antihypertensives, of which Diuril is one) might help preserve bone structure at the same time that it reduces blood pressure because it tends to reduce the amount of calcium excreted in the urine. With ACE (anticholinesterase) inhibitors, another class of antihypertensive medications, cough was two to three times more common in women than in men. Women given a calcium channel blocker (still another class) are more likely than men to develop swelling of their ankles and legs. Men are less responsive than women to the category of antihypertensives that work by blocking the effects of the sympathetic nervous system on the heart. And last but certainly not least, an important side effect of many antihypertensive drugs for men is sexual dysfunction, which has really not been studied adequately in women.

Coronary Artery Disease

Until very recently, doctors and patients alike thought that coronary artery disease (CAD)* affected only middle-age men. Most women still fear they will die of breast cancer and are aware of the importance of regular testing and early detection for survival. What they don't know is that cardiovascular disease kills more women than all cancers combined and that for all of us—both men and women—CAD is the most important of all the illnesses that threaten our lives.

The fact is that half a million American women die each year of cardiovascular disease. Half of them die of CAD, and 100,000 of those

---

* Coronary artery disease is the illness in which a combination of cholesterol, calcium, clot, and other elements called *plaque* builds up inside the coronary arteries, narrowing the passageway for blood to reach and nourish the heart muscle. If the obstruction is too great, part of the heart muscle dies. This is called a heart attack (or a myocardial infarction).

deaths are premature. Alarmed by these statistics, women have begun urging doctors to pay more attention to their potential for heart disease. My own introduction to the issue came from Carol Colman, the medical journalist who walked into my office one day nine years ago and asked me to help her research and write a book about women and CAD. I wondered why she thought this necessary; what, I asked, was so different about CAD in women? It happened that Carol's mother, who eventually died of CAD, had been misdiagnosed and inaccurately treated by physicians. Carol was convinced that women experienced the disease differently than men, and that doctors in general believed (wrongly) that CAD was not a significant problem in women. Even if women *had* CAD, doctors thought, it was not as serious for them, as they were protected by their hormones in a way that men were not. Carol believed that her mother's illness and subsequent death could have been prevented, and she was determined that other women should not suffer the same fate.

WHAT IS CORONARY ARTERY DISEASE?

Like all organs, the heart muscle is fed by arteries that supply it with the blood it needs for work and survival. CAD results when a waxy substance called *plaque* (composed of cholesterol, clots, and other debris) accumulates in the arteries that supply the heart. Plaque narrows the inner diameter or *lumen* of the artery, and the flow of blood diminishes. If not enough blood reaches the heart tissue to supply it with the energy it needs, a portion of it dies. This is a heart attack, or *myocardial infarction*.

Several things besides plaque can cause a heart attack as well. If the surface of the plaque ruptures, a clot can form at the site of the break, further decreasing the space through which blood can pass. In other cases, the coronary artery itself contracts, narrowing the artery and restricting the blood flow to the heart. A critical degree of coronary artery constriction can be fatal in patients with other complicating factors: among these are cocaine (a powerful coronary artery vasoconstrictor) and sudden estrogen deficiency in women (estrogen helps keep coronary arteries dilated and able to bring critical amounts of blood to the heart muscle).

DO WOMEN AND MEN EXPERIENCE CAD IN THE SAME WAY?

Until recently, doctors believed that the actual experience of CAD was the same in both sexes. They believed that the symptoms of the illness, the factors that make some people more susceptible than others (risk factors), the way the disease is experienced over time (its clinical course), and the chances for recovery and survival (outcome) were similar if not identical for both men and women. (As I have said, this was because virtually all research on CAD had been done on men, and doctors were taught that the data could be applied to women without modification.) At the same time, and probably due to limited data about the illness in women, doctors (and many patients) believed that women didn't get CAD until they were very old, and that when they did, the illness was milder than in men. Research done over the last ten years has taught us the opposite, that CAD is more lethal for females who suffer a heart attack (particularly those under fifty) than for males. And current gender-specific research on CAD in women has turned up a number of important findings.

RISK FACTORS

The risk factors and warning signs for CAD are generally the same for women as they are for men, but there are also important differences.

SERUM LIPID LEVEL: The fat in food cannot be used by the body until it has been processed by the liver and absorbed by the intestine. As a result of this process, several products of the fats we eat are carried in the blood. The principal ones are cholesterol and triglycerides. Cholesterol itself can be broken down into "bad" cholesterol or low-density lipoprotein (LDL), which is the type of fat that is deposited in the walls of arteries and is one of the principal ingredients of plaque. The other type is "good" cholesterol or high-density lipoprotein (HDL), which helps *prevent* plaque from forming. The two together are measured in the laboratory from a patient's blood sample as total cholesterol (TC).

Men and women have different optimal levels of serum fats or lipids. While men can have HDL levels as low as 35 mg/dL of blood, women begin to have increased risk for CAD below levels of 45 mg/dL. HDL levels are particularly important in predicting resistance—or susceptibility—to heart disease in women: values below 30 are a matter for serious concern and treatment. Values above 60 mg/dL, on the other hand, are considered a *protection* against risk for CAD. For men, triglyceride levels can go as high as 400 mg/dL of blood without an increased risk of CAD; for women, optimal levels are under 200.

DIABETES: Diabetes is an important risk factor for both sexes for cardiovascular disease, especially CAD. It is more dangerous for women, however, as diabetes in women increases the risk of CAD four- to sixfold, even if a woman is young and/or premenopausal. In diabetic men, the risk of CAD is doubled.

Diabetes is important in other respects for cardiac patients of both sexes. Because diabetes affects and destroys nervous tissue, diabetic patients may not be warned by chest pain that they are having a heart attack, or that the supply of blood to their heart muscle is dangerously low. Men and women with diabetes, and their doctors, should take care to be alert to the signs and symptoms of CAD.

AGE: Both men and women are more susceptible to CAD as they age. In general, though, the symptoms and signs of CAD begin to be apparent in men by the time they are thirty-five; in women, the disease is usually not symptomatic until they are about forty-five. Researchers have recently described a group of women between the ages of twenty and fifty with myocardial infarctions who did very poorly; they died twice as often in the hospital as did men of the same age. As is so often the case, these observations push us to reconsider our model of how heart attacks happen. The younger women who have heart attacks may suffer them because they have an abnormally high tendency to form blood clots in their vessels, including their coronary arteries, or because they have an exaggerated tendency to go into spasm, usually, but not always, because they are smokers. It is also probable that instead of rupturing, the plaque in the coronary arteries of these women erodes and attracts material that forms a clot that occludes the vessel.

HYPERTENSION: Men and women have different consequences of high blood pressure, although for both it is a significant risk factor for CAD. Before menopause, women's blood pressure is lower than that of same-age men, but as women age, their blood pressure increases at a faster rate than that of men. As I have explained, male and female hearts respond differently to hypertension: the left ventricle, which pumps blood out of the heart to supply the entire body, has a different pattern of enlargement in the two sexes. This difference is the result of hormones—it disappears in castrated rats with high blood pressure. We do not yet know if this information will lead to treating hypertension in humans with hormone therapy.

OBESITY: Being 30 percent over ideal body weight increases the risk of both sexes for CAD. Men have greater risk than women at any given weight, however, because most of their fat is in the abdominal region, while women tend to collect excess fat in the buttocks and thighs. Abdominal fat is metabolized more actively in the liver than fat in other areas of the body, and it produces higher levels of serum cholesterol and triglycerides. Postmenopausal women, however, tend to resemble men in the way their fat is distributed. As they gain weight, their waistlines thicken, and they become more apple-shaped rather than pear-shaped. An important study of the effects of post-menopausal HRT in reducing women's risk factors for CAD established that HRT seemed to slow weight gain and reduce the dangerous accumulation of fat around the abdomen. Obesity in general seems to be a risk factor for women. Investigators at Harvard who conducted a long-term study of a population of nurses observed that women with the lowest body mass index have the lowest probability of developing CAD. This finding is corroborated by studies in monkeys, which have shown that those fed the least amount of calories compatible with good nutrition lived the longest.

FAMILY HISTORY: Having a first-degree relative (mother, father, sister, or brother) who dies of CAD before the age of fifty-five increases the risk for CAD in both men and women. For women, the risk is more serious if the relative is female. Such women should be evaluated each year for the signs of CAD; even children of families with a strong history of CAD should have their serum lipids monitored. No matter how young the patient, higher-than-normal levels of lipids should be aggressively treated with diet and exercise.

MENOPAUSAL STATE: While menopause is often blamed for (and can be the cause of) a whole host of ills, it does not seem to put aging women at increased risk for CAD. Risk for CAD in both men and women normally increases with age and increases still further if a person smokes, but menopause itself does not make women uniquely vulnerable.

LIFESTYLE RISK FACTORS

SMOKING: Of all the things we voluntarily do that cause illness, smoking is the most lethal. Even one cigarette a day increases risk for both sexes. This fact makes it particularly dismaying to read that the greatest numbers of new smokers are teenage girls. Early smoking is particularly harmful for girls, as it actually stunts the growth of their lungs. Boys, on the other hand, seem able to smoke with greater impunity; unlike girl smokers, boy smokers do not have smaller lung volumes than their nonsmoking peers. Severe CAD in young women (under the age of forty) is almost always associated with smoking.

LACK OF EXERCISE: Unfortunately from the standpoint of our physical fitness, the tremendous advances in science and technology over the past century have provided Americans with an increasing amount of leisure time and freedom from physical labor. The result is an epidemic of obesity: 97 million Americans are overweight, and the number has doubled over the last thirty-five years.

Exercise lessens the amount of sympathetic nervous system input to the heart, which in turn lowers heart rate, even at rest; exercise lowers blood pressure and causes the heart muscle to contract less vigorously with each beat. It doesn't take much exercise to reduce the risk for CAD dramatically: just walking briskly for forty minutes a day three times a week can reduce the risk by 40 percent!

Stress: For both men and women, stress can literally be lethal. Some kinds of stress can be productive and health giving: a healthy sense of competitiveness, a sense of urgency to achieve, and a willingness to volunteer and excel at work are all useful and even desirable human traits. *The kind of stress that kills is unique: it is best described as the emotional reaction that the sufferer has to problems that cause intense pain and difficulty and that apparently cannot be solved or relieved.*

Many men are convinced that modern women have heart attacks because a growing number of them are working outside the home, which increases their stress levels. In fact, that is not the case at all. The Framingham Heart Study, one of the classic longitudinal studies (a study done over a relatively long period of time on the same group of patients) of CAD in both men and women, has shown that the women at lowest risk for CAD are those who find their work rewarding and are unmarried with no children.[2] Women in what the Framingham investigators call "pink collar" jobs, who find their work unrewarding emotionally and/or financially, are at higher risk for CAD, while women in unrewarding jobs with primary responsibility for young children or infirm adults are at the highest risk of all. A study of married couples at a Volvo plant in Sweden found that when men and women arrived home, women's blood pressure and heart rates rose as they crossed the threshold, while men's fell![3]

Both men and women, when faced with problems that cause them significant emotional duress and anxiety, experience an increase in the input of the sympathetic nervous system to the heart: their heart rates and blood pressure rise. If the stress is chronic, the adrenal glands begin to manufacture cortisol to counter the effects of prolonged stress on the body. While it may mitigate agitation in response to stress, cortisol also pushes blood pressure up and adversely affects the body's metabolism. In fact, the emotion most commonly associated with a heart attack is a sense of pervasive hopelessness, which is also a common feature of long-standing stress. When I ask patients who have suffered a heart attack, "How do you think this happened to you?" every single one has answered, "I have been under a great deal of stress over the past few weeks/months/years."

USE OF RECREATIONAL DRUGS: Although many patients refuse to talk about it, the use of illicit drugs is quite common. Cocaine is a particularly lethal substance for *both* men and women: it produces spasm of the coronary arteries (as well as other arteries, including those that supply blood to the brain). It can accelerate and/or destabilize the rhythm of the heart, producing stroke, heart attack, or sudden cardiac death even in very young, healthy individuals—including superbly fit athletes. Cocaine users would do well to remember that a person can often have CAD, even to an advanced degree, without symptoms. In addition to the drug's damaging addictive properties, cocaine can constrict arteries that are already partially occluded by plaque, with catastrophic consequences.

TESTING FOR CAD

The most common test for CAD is the standard stress test. In this test, the patient is attached to monitoring leads, which record heartbeat, and to a blood pressure cuff, which measures blood pressure. The patient then walks on a treadmill as the incline and the speed are slowly increased, raising the heart rate to the maximum predicted safe value for his or her sex and age. The physician is able to tell from the changes (or absence of changes) in the ECG and blood pressure whether the heart is equal to the work it is being asked to do. While this kind of test is *specific* (accurately diagnosing a given kind of disease) and *sensitive* (actually detecting the presence of CAD) for men, it is neither specific nor sensitive enough for women and should not be used to screen for CAD in females.

ECGs in women are more likely to change during the course of a treadmill test even when the heart is actually quite healthy and is meeting the demands imposed on it (a false positive). Doctors do not know the reason for the unacceptably high incidence of false positives on treadmill tests in women. Women are more accurately tested with the stress echocardiogram, in which an ultrasound probe captures an image of the heart's motion at rest and again at peak exercise. If the test shows that the heart motion is abnormal (a segment of the muscle moves weakly, doesn't move at all, or paradoxically expands when the rest of the heart is contracting), the probability of CAD is extremely high.

Another kind of test uses radioactive tracers to assess the flow of blood to the heart during rest and exercise; it is equally accurate in men and women. But large breasts can interfere with the testing process; women with large breasts must be carefully positioned and the test evaluated by experts to make sure that the patient is not misdiagnosed with heart trouble when the problem is poorly transmitted signals.

CLINICAL SYMPTOMS OF A HEART ATTACK

The classic symptoms of a heart attack are a sensation of burning pain or of pressure (sometimes tremendous pressure) in the center of the chest. It may radiate down the left arm or down both arms and into the neck and jaw. For fully 20 percent of women with heart attacks, however, the symptoms are quite different: pain in the upper abdomen or back, intense shortness of breath, nausea, and profuse sweating. Such women may be misdiagnosed as having indigestion or a gallbladder attack. Their shortness of breath may be interpreted as an anxiety attack; many women, particularly if they are young, are sent home from emergency rooms with Mylanta and Valium, only to return in much more serious condition or when it is too late to help them.

OUTCOME OF A FIRST HEART ATTACK

The first heart attack is much more dangerous for women than for men. Contrary to the popular belief that CAD is more serious in men, studies show that 39 percent of women will die within the first weeks after their first heart attack, as compared with 31 percent of men. Women are also more likely than men to have a second attack within the following few years. Women who do survive are less likely than men to be able to return to their normal pre-attack lifestyles and are less likely to resume sexual activity. More females than males suffer from depression after a myocardial infarction (which may simply reflect the higher incidence of depression in women in the general population). A recent study reported that men with CAD had a better mood and outlook three years after their heart attack, but that women had better levels of physical recovery. The doctors who did this study felt that most of the men had a greater social support system than most of the women. While having a lot of help might keep the patient's mood up, it might also make him more dependent and less likely to do the work needed for a return to full strength and health. On the other hand, a lack of friends and family to help care for the patient who is recovering from a heart attack might make her more susceptible to depression. Another interesting outcome of this study is that in both sexes recovery, both physical and emotional, seemed to plateau in year three after the heart attack. The researchers urged doctors and the families of heart attack victims to continue their efforts to restore patients to better levels of emotional and physical health for longer than just a few months.

Do Physicians Give Men and Women with Symptoms of CAD the Same Treatment?

As I pointed out in the beginning of this chapter, the unfortunate and undeniable fact is that men and women are still being treated differently by their doctors for the same diseases. This isn't true only of heart disease: across the board, women are treated more conservatively than men for their illnesses. A woman with end-stage kidney disease, for example, is less likely than a man to get a kidney transplant. As disturbing as this was when it was pointed out for the first time in the late 1980s, it was more upsetting to read a 1999 paper by Kevin Schulman and his colleagues at Georgetown University College of Medicine indicating that even when patients with cardiac symptoms told identical stories, both their race *and* their sex influenced physicians' decisions about whether to send them on for further testing.[4] Black women were significantly less likely than white men to be referred for cardiac catheterization tests. The difference in the way physicians treat the two sexes was most marked for black women, who were the least likely to be sent on for definitive diagnosis on the basis of their histories. In addition, women are often offered only medication for their CAD, while men are offered *thrombolytic therapy* (clot-busting therapy that can open an occluded, or blocked, coronary artery if performed promptly after a heart attack) and *angioplasty* (a procedure in which a catheter, a thin tube, is inserted via an artery into the occluded coronary artery and a balloon at the catheter tip is inflated at the point of obstruction, compressing the obstructing plaque against the arterial wall). Several refinements and variations on the angioplasty procedure are now available. In some the plaque is vaporized by a laser beam and the fragments are harmlessly dispersed downstream from the point of obstruction. Stenting—or propping the artery open with a permanent tube—can be introduced to prevent reocclusion, and local radiation can prevent a new obstruction at the same site.

Open-heart surgery is also recommended more often for men. Even when women do have this kind of surgery, cardiac surgeons make different decisions: in female patients, surgeons less frequently choose the internal mammary artery for bypass of the obstructed site, even though it is superior to a vein because it is less likely to become occluded in the months and years after surgery. Studies from the United Kingdom and Israel as well as the United States have noted many of these discrepancies in the care of men and women with CAD. After citing them, the investigators consistently make the same statement: "Reasons for these differences remain obscure."

In 1992 the Council on Ethical and Judicial Affairs of the American Medical Association published an important paper warning physicians that these striking differences in the way men and women were treated—not only for CAD, but across the board—reflected genuine bias about what care men and women could endure and should have.[5] Whether the discrepancies are due more to the reluctance of women to accept more aggressive choices for treatment, or to physicians regarding women as less valuable than men (an opinion speculated on by the council in its landmark statement), or to an effort to protect women is unknown at this point.

If physicians do fear treating illnesses in women aggressively, such fears are unwarranted. Data from the National Heart, Lung, and Blood Institute, which collected the results of angioplasty procedures over a period of years and compared the results in men and women, showed that while women had a slightly higher mortality rate (2 percent higher), survival was at least 95 percent in both sexes. Although women had a higher mortality when they underwent coronary artery bypass grafting, this was because they were generally older and sicker than men, with more coexisting diseases, at the time of the surgery. If women with CAD are diagnosed early on and are referred promptly for bypass when appropriate, they do as well as men in the sophisticated hospitals that perform these procedures frequently.

CARDIAC REHABILITATION

The limited data on gender differences in CAD recovery programs tell us what we might expect, that although physicians refer fewer female heart attack survivors (than males) to such programs women tend to participate in them as enthusiastically as men and to realize as many benefits from them.

In summary, cardiovascular disease is the chief killer of both men and women in the United States; not only are women not exempt from the disease, it is more severe in them, and women are more likely than men to die of their first heart attack. While men's death rate from CAD is declining, women's is not. Physicians are just beginning to be aware that the risk factors, clinical presentation, testing modalities, therapeutic choices, and consequences of CAD are not identical in men and women. In spite of scientists' expanding understanding of these differences, a recent study revealed that many physicians do not counsel women patients, even when they are over sixty, about techniques to reduce their risk for CAD and omit essential testing to assess whether they have it or are at high risk for acquiring it. Men and women alike should know how to assess their risk for CAD and should be aware of the range of therapeutic options that are available in order to make an informed decision about treatment and rehabilitation. Finally, the entire community of women, as well as the physicians who care for them, should be aware of the regrettable tendency of doctors to minimize the cardiac complaints of women, attributing them to depression or hysteria. Such gender prejudice often results in late diagnosis of CAD, when it is far advanced and survival is less likely. Significant numbers of women, particularly young women, are sent out of emergency rooms with a diagnosis of panic disorder or hysteria, then go on to die from undiagnosed CAD. Prompt and accurate diagnosis and effective treatment of this, the chief killer of adults in this country, is the right of both men and women.

WHAT DOES THE NEW SCIENCE MEAN FOR YOU?

As a woman, how can I be sure that my doctor isn't dismissing my complaints or treating my heart disease less aggressively than is warranted?

Unfortunately, as we've seen in this chapter, the odds are still against women receiving a prompt, accurate diagnosis and aggressive, optimal care for heart disease. To be an effective advocate for yourself under these circumstances, be sure to get organized before you see your doctor. Make a list of your complaints and the questions to which you need answers. If you have a specific problem, include a description of when it began, exactly what it feels like, what causes it, how long it lasts, and what makes it better or worse. Put together an orderly story that's as accurate as you can make it. Keep it simple, concise, and clear.

If your doctor dismisses your complaints out of hand as psychosomatic and refuses to send you for diagnostic testing, challenge her. If she can't collaborate with you to find out whether your symptoms indicate heart disease, she's not useful to you. Continuing to be her patient may literally cost you your life, or at least valuable time before a correct diagnosis is made.

When you are given a treatment plan, question it very carefully, making sure you understand what medications you are being offered and how they are expected to work.

If I have an arrhythmia, what should I expect my doctor to know about the **normal** *differences between my heart and circulation and a man's?*

Because the heart's electrical system differs between men and women, your heart rate will be faster than a man's, and your electrocardiogram will differ in some respects as well. You are more likely to *perceive* that you are having occasional extra beats of your heart, without their necessarily being more frequent than is normal. Nevertheless, you are more likely to develop long runs of rapid heart rates, particularly just before or on the first day of your menstrual period.

If you have been diagnosed with an arrhythmia, don't be shy about telling your doctor that your bursts of rapid heart rate (the most common kind of this arrhythmia is called *paroxysmal atrial tachycardia*, by the way) are likely to occur just before you have your menstrual period. You are *not* imagining it—it's due to the sudden drop-off of available estrogen during this time in your cycle. Using a low-dose estrogen patch during these few vulnerable days is a good way to eliminate this problem (and may also take care of your "menstrual migraine"—the headache many women experience during these low-estrogen days).

If you are perimenopausal (your menstrual periods have not stopped but now occur irregularly, and you experience some of the symptoms of menopause like hot flashes or difficulty sleeping) and you are suddenly experiencing bursts of palpitations and even longer runs of rapid heart rate, you need to find out whether they are a sign of heart disease and ask your doctor for appropriate diagnostic testing. Most likely, though, they are due to wildly fluctuating levels of estrogen—sometimes very high and at other times very low. Taking an oral contraceptive pill is an excellent way to smooth out these irregularities until you reach true menopause and your menstrual periods stop altogether.

If you are given a medication to control extra heartbeats, *ask your doctor if the medicine was tested for safety in women!* It's unlikely that your doctor will know the answer, but women are unquestionably more likely to develop a potentially fatal arrhythmia when given certain drugs. If, after taking it, you feel no relief or even an increase in symptoms, consult your physician at once.

Should I ask my doctor to test my thyroid gland periodically to make sure it is not underactive?

Women have "stiffer" hearts than men as they age, because older female hearts have more connective tissue than younger ones.

Hypothyroidism accelerates this "stiffening" process. Restoring the thyroid gland's activity to normal is important if you have any signs of congestive heart failure (shortness of breath, rapid heart rates on minimal exertion that take a long time to return to normal, and/or swollen ankles). Ask your doctor to test your levels of *thyroid-stimulating hormone* and *circulating thyroid hormone*. If the tests show an underactive gland, small doses of thyroid replacement therapy can help lower cholesterol, control weight, relieve fatigue, and prevent the development of the "stiff" heart that makes relaxation of the heart muscle between beats more difficult and makes the heart function less efficiently.

Should I be worried about high blood pressure? What's the best gender-specific treatment for me if it develops?

Before menopause most women are protected from high blood pressure, but after sixty more women than men have hypertension. The consequences are somewhat different for the two sexes.

Ask your doctor to take your blood pressure in both arms and, if the first value(s) are high, several times during the examination. Don't underestimate the difficulty of getting a good reading: if your heart rate is slow and the measurement is made too quickly, the reading may not be accurate.

For most women with high blood pressure, doctors prescribe a kind of medication called a beta-blocker, an anti-anxiety drug, as a first choice. Not only does this choice reflect a conviction that a woman's out-of-control emotions are causing her high blood pressure, but such drugs are more expensive than other antihypertensive medicines. Beta-blockers also have significant side effects in some patients: they tend to raise cholesterol levels and may put you at risk for asthma and depression (or at least unusual feelings of tiredness). A simple diuretic (or water pill) might be reasonable to try first. Another bonus of the diuretics is that they tend to preserve bone mass (by reducing the amount of calcium secreted in the urine).

After about three months, your blood pressure may go up again. Have your doctor adjust your medication and/or change the kind that you are taking.

If you develop high blood pressure while you are taking an oral contraceptive, stop taking it! Particularly if there is a history of high blood pressure in your family, ask your doctor for one of the tricyclic formula pills, which produce hypertension less frequently than other kinds of oral contraceptives.

Various kinds of antihypertensive medications are more likely to produce side effects in women, who are more likely to develop a cough on an ACE inhibitor and swelling of the ankles and feet on a calcium channel blocker.

Sexual dysfunction as a result of antihypertensive medicine has been well studied in men but not in women. If you notice any change in libido, in your ability to achieve orgasm, or in the intensity of your orgasm, ask your doctor to change your drug. By the way, one of the little-known consequences of diuretic therapy in women is that it may dry the vaginal lining and make intercourse uncomfortable. (Antihistamines can do the same thing.)

As a woman, what are the most important things I have to know about coronary artery disease?

There are very important differences between men and women in virtually every aspect of the experience of CAD.

- Diabetes is probably the most important risk factor of all for a woman; it removes any protection she has by virtue of her age or premenopausal state.
- Symptoms of an acute heart attack in one out of five women are not classic but involve epigastric pain, excessive sweating, and extreme shortness of breath.
- The optimal noninvasive testing modality (that doesn't involve a radioactive tracer) for women is a stress echocardiogram; a simple treadmill test is neither specific nor sensitive enough in females to make it worth doing.
- After a myocardial infarction, women are much less likely than men to receive optimal therapy, which should include a beta-blocker, ACE inhibitor, an aggressive lowering of LDL cholesterol levels

to below 100 mg/dL, and a daily aspirin. *A low HDL (below 45) should be aggressively treated in women;* as a risk factor, it has much more serious prognostic implications for women than for men.

- Recent data suggest that *women with established coronary artery disease should not be started on hormone replacement therapy.* But women who were on HRT *before* they developed CAD can safely continue it. These recommendations may change as data from the Women's Health Initiative, an ongoing study supported by the National Heart, Lung, and Blood Institute of the NIH, accumulate and are reported to physicians.

- The waist-hip ratio is a more accurate indicator of risk for CAD than the body mass index. Be sure to ask your doctor to measure it for you, and if you have to lose weight, follow its improvement. (It should be 0.8 or less.)

- JoAnn Manson, who is now supervising the Nurses' Health Study, points out that *correcting poor lifestyle habits can lower the incidence of coronary artery disease in both sexes by 83 percent!* Stop smoking (even one cigarette a day increases risk), pursue a reasonable and *consistent* exercise program, and pay particular attention to reducing stress in your life. As a woman, once you've had a heart attack, you are less likely than a man to be referred to a cardiac rehabilitation program, which is very important in returning you to full function. You are also more likely to be significantly depressed than a man and are less likely to return to your former level of activity, particularly to your pre–heart attack level of sexual activity. Ask your doctor to help put you in and keep you in an aggressive campaign to regain your health and confidence.

CHAPTER 6

The Immune System

WE EXIST IN a hostile universe, surrounded by enemies of all sizes and kinds that we can easily identify, and we defend ourselves against them well before they even make contact with our bodies. There are other enemies, though, that we can't see; they invade our bodies, usually without our even being aware of it. We eat them, breathe them in; some even enter through a cut in our skin. Thousands of encounters with hostile agents take place within us every day. Remarkably, we are so insulated from them that we're completely unaware of the fact that our defenses meet and conquer them. Our survival against these invisible enemies—the toxins, bacteria, and viruses that threaten our health—depends on a complex, integrated array of defenses called the immune system. It is our body's police force, possessed of thousands of weapons from which to choose, each of which helps to address and conquer a specific threat. The immune system is so effective that we can—and do—overcome many infections and destroy many foreign substances without the help of medicines. Every so often, though, we become all too aware that our body is fighting a powerful enemy. Fever, aching muscles, rashes—a hundred miseries tell us that a big battle is being waged.

The immune system depends on the perfectly orchestrated interplay among an enormous number of molecules produced by the many different kinds of cells that defend us. It is amazing that most of the time it is so stable, predictable, and effective, given the many opportunities for things to go wrong. And sometimes they do.

Probably the most important task the immune system has to master is to distinguish "self" from "nonself." The ability to make this distinction is called tolerance, and it is programmed into the cells that defend us from their earliest existence. When tolerance is lost or missing, these cells begin to attack our own tissues. This is the basis for what doctors call *autoimmune disease,* like systemic lupus erythematosus and rheumatoid arthritis. Most but not all of these diseases are more common in women than in men.

One of the great mysteries that scientists have yet to solve is why the body sometimes attacks its own tissue as though it were an enemy. Autoimmune diseases are among the least well understood—and as a result, they resist our best efforts to cure them. Chronic fatigue syndrome, fibromyalgia—these are diseases that often follow a major, poorly characterized illness, probably caused by a viral agent, and that plague patients for years after the infection is "over" and the acute sickness subsides. Poor Job, with his succession of trials, no doubt had to bear an autoimmune disease as one of his torments. The Book of Job is a wonderful one for a sick person—as well as a physician—to read: the poor afflicted patient laments the state of his skin; he is covered with boils from his scalp to the soles of his feet—a scourge that he doesn't understand, can't relieve, and drives him to despair. The intelligence and dignity with which he chides the God who has allowed him to be so relentlessly, interminably afflicted are remarkable. Perhaps no one has given voice to the question "why me, Lord?" as brilliantly—or movingly—as Job.

HOW THE IMMUNE SYSTEM WORKS

The body protects itself against invaders in two ways. The first is called the *innate immune system.* Its components don't require special tailoring to repulse or destroy toxic agents: they are always there and ready as a first line of defense. Some are simply physical barriers to invaders, like the skin, or the mucus in our respiratory passages. Others are chemicals that the body keeps on hand as first responders to a foreign bacteria or poison.*

The second way the body protects itself is much more specific; in what is called the *adaptive immune system*, it mobilizes in response to an individual, unique invader. This system depends on the work of special cells, called leukocytes, that originate from multipotential ancestors called stem cells. Stem cells are produced from our earliest existence: first in the yolk sac that provides the first nourishment for the fertilized ovum, then in the liver, and then, as soon as the skeleton is formed, within the bone marrow. Some descendants of the stem cells continue to develop in the bone marrow (called granulocytes). Others migrate to mature in our lymph nodes (called B lymphocytes or B cells and natural killer cells) or in the thymus gland† (these are called T lymphocytes or T cells). Finally, there is a group of leukocytes that is specially adapted for presenting foreign material from invaders to other cells of the immune system; these are called specialized antigen presenting cells.

Each class of cells in the adaptive immune system participates in unique ways to challenge and defeat an enemy. Like the components of an army, the granulocytes, the specialized antigen-presenting cells, and the lymphocytes all have different tasks to do, all of which contribute to winning the war. The essential task, though, is to recognize an enemy and construct a response that destroys it. Destruction is achieved either through a direct attack by a defending cell or through a series of maneuvers involving a complex molecule produced by a B cell called an antibody. Antibodies attach to the enemy and either neutralize its ability to harm us or prepare it for destruction by other cells and/or chemicals in the arsenal of the immune system.

---

* Among these chemicals are *chemokines*, which cause defending white cells, or leukocytes, to migrate to the toxic agent or substance, and *cytokines*, which prime the leukocytes for attack.

† The thymus is a gland that forms in the chest during development. It partially disappears at puberty, but rudiments of it remain throughout our life. The minimizing of the thymus gland appears to be regulated by testosterone.

Specialized Antigen-Presenting Cells

The specialized antigen-presenting cells are the immune army's foot soldiers: they are a first line of defense against an invader. When such a cell meets an enemy, it consumes and digests it. It then moves pieces of the enemy's foreign proteins (called antigens), like trophies of the encounter, up to its own surface. This foot soldier then brings its antigen-trophy (a little like the scalp of an enemy) to the T cell for further action. Before it does so, however, special molecules on the surface of the antigen-presenting cell called human leukocyte antigens (HLA) perform an essential function: they mark our own cells as "self" with identifiers as individual as fingerprints, allowing our immune system to recognize them and let them pass unchallenged throughout the body.

The foot soldier then presents the antigen to a T cell so that the T cell can recognize a combination of the HLA molecule and the antigen.* The foot soldier, in effect, has become a policeman, bringing a criminal to a judge—in this case, the T cell—for disposition. Like patrolmen on duty, specialized antigen-presenting cells are stationed everywhere in the body that invaders are particularly likely to enter.

T Cells

The T cells (so named because they mature in the thymus gland) are the strategists in this war, the elements in the immune system that determine, among other things, how the invader is to be destroyed. The T cell has a special docking place on its surface into which the specialized antigen-presenting cell can lock its trophy. This place is called the T cell receptor (TCR).† One way of classifying T cells is by the kinds of receptors they have. Each type has one of two different kinds of special molecules that are associated with the TCR; one is called CD4 and the other is called CD8.

---

* There are two major classes of genes that make these HLA molecules, and within each class further variations are possible (six genes in class I and ten in class II).

† The TCR is so cunningly fashioned that it will not recognize any of our own proteins as enemy; the gene that governs its production is fixed and cannot change.

CD8 T cells are involved in dampening or suppressing some aspects of the immune process, and in other instances they directly attack and destroy infected cells. For this reason, they are also called suppressor or cytotoxic T cells.

In general (but not always), CD4 positive T cells (T4 cells) "help" or intensify the immune process and thus are called helper cells. Helper cells are necessary to help the B cell produce antibodies against most of the antigens it meets. T4 cells respond only to antigens bound to class II HLA molecules, and T cells associated with CD8 (T8 cells) only to class I.

Women, who have more intense immune systems than men, also have more CD4 lymphocytes. CD4 T cells are further divided into two types, depending on the type of chemicals (cytokines) they produce when they fight off invaders. One subset of T4 cells, called T_H1, makes cytokines that promote inflammation in response to an invader; the other subset, called T_H2, produces a set of cytokines that promote the production of antibodies by B cells. The two types of cells within the CD4 T cell population cross-regulate each other. Women are more likely than men to mount a T_H1 response to invaders— except during pregnancy, when a T_H2 response prevails. This guarantees a vigorous response to infection and a dampening of the body's response to alien invasion, which protects the fetus carrying molecules patterned after its father, to which the mother's immune system might otherwise react.

This unique, sex-determined capability of the immune system explains why in animal experiments females have less severe viral infections, since viruses are destroyed by a brisk inflammatory response. On the other hand, if a virus invades the central nervous system, females are more likely to have damage, because the inflammatory response they mount is more intense than that of males.

Women's more vigorous immune system may well be the result of evolutionary selection. Women are the custodians of the family and as such are usually the ones assigned to nursing the sick members of that family (particularly the youngest) back to health. It's probable that women with ineffective defenses against contagious diseases died out and those best equipped to defend against contagious illness survived.

B Cells

B cells work differently from T cells. They are like the special forces of an army, in that they mount very efficient defenses against an enemy and then remember the enemy so that when it comes again, their defenses against it are already developed and primed to defeat it. Each B cell is equipped to make a uniquely configured molecule (called an antibody), which is capable of attaching to a specific antigen. An antibody is much like a lock into which a particular key, the antigen, can fit. Once it combines with the antigen, the B cell is "switched on" and begins to make copies of itself.

Each time a B cell divides to make two daughter cells (or clones of itself), it rearranges its genetic equipment so that the antibody it makes becomes more and more specific for the antigen it is fighting; eventually, the cloned daughter cells that result make a very precisely fitting antibody. The stronger the bond between the antibodies the B cell produces and the antigen, the more likely it is that the B cell will survive. The daughter cells that finally result from this process, therefore, have extraordinary specificity for the attacker and are very efficient in destroying it.

In most cases, B cells need the help of T cells to produce effective and fine-tuned antibodies. But some antigens can be attacked by B cell antibodies without the help of T cells. These antibodies are less precisely specialized and so can react with many antigens in addition to the offending agent. Because they are so promiscuous, as it were, these less specific antibodies act against our own tissue, and at least for a short while, they can produce symptoms characteristic of an autoimmune disease.

Granulocytes

The granulocytes function as mop-up and support troops. They produce inflammation in the tissues, which helps to eliminate invaders. After an invader has been identified and its component parts have been used to mobilize resistance from the immune system, the granulocytes infiltrate the battlefield to ingest and destroy targeted antigens that have been coated with antibodies or other elements of the immune system. There are several kinds of granulocytes, each category designed to be particularly effective against a particular kind of invader. Special cells in this group work against bacteria, others work against parasites like worms, and still others are involved in allergic responses.

The most abundant (over 70 percent) of the circulating granulocytes are called *polymorphonuclear leukocytes.* They patrol the bloodstream until they sense (through chemicals released in the blood vessels at the site of invasion) an enemy: they attach to the blood vessel wall and migrate into the surrounding tissue, where they release their granules (just as a soldier fires grenades and bullets at the enemy); these granules not only kill the enemy but can cause actual damage to infected tissue.

Some data in animal experiments show important differences in the activity of granulocytes between males and females. The activities of these cells, under different circumstances and even in the same tissues, vary as a function of gender. For example, anesthetizing male rats makes their granulocytes inactive, while those of female rats continue to function. The response to a challenge by alcohol or by a poison produced by certain bacteria called an endotoxin is more vigorous in female rats of reproductive age than it is in males or in prepubescent and postreproductive-age female rats. Again, this kind of defense may be evolutionary in origin.

The cells of the immune system are great travelers; they have to be so that they can encounter the enemy wherever it invades. Scientists estimate that the average lymphocyte spends only about thirty minutes in the bloodstream during each cycle it makes around the body; the rest of the time it is moving through tissues on patrol for enemies. The cells involved in the immune process concentrate at specialized sites in areas where the enemy makes its first entry into the body: the digestive tract, the respiratory tract, and if the enemy has invaded the bloodstream, the spleen. If invading organisms breach initial defenses and invade tissue, the local lymph nodes respond to dispose of them. These specialized areas of tissue are like equipment and personnel-laden supply stations for a battlefield's front line, where all the elements needed for a maximum immune response are concentrated.

AUTOIMMUNE DISEASES

What Are They?

The power of the immune system is potentially devastating; it is fine-tuned to destroy whatever it sees as alien. But when it loses the vitally important ability to distinguish between our own tissue and a foreign substance or invading enemy, the result is an autoimmune disease. The assault can be due to a general breakdown in the function of T and B cells, or it can involve a *specific erroneous response to a particular antigen*. In the first instance, as in systemic lupus erythematosus, the immune system attacks a whole variety of the patient's tissues. The result is widespread destruction: the lupus patient can exhibit fever, rash, hair loss, arthritis, inflammation of the thin sacs of protective tissue that cover the lungs and heart, kidney failure, blood disorders, and inflammation of the brain all at the same time. This kind of generalized attack, which produces such devastation, has inspired the medical term *protean manifestations of disease,* after the Greek god Proteus, who could assume many different forms and thus evade recognition. In the second instance, the treatment or response to a single antigen goes wrong and affects only one tissue (like the kind of damage to nerves that follows a specific gastrointestinal infection by the organism called *Campylobacter jejuni,* or like the destruction of the insulin-producing cells of the pancreas that causes type 1 diabetes).

There are several phenomena that seem to activate autoimmune disorders. Sometimes an environmental trigger seems to be the culprit, for example, an autoimmune disease called pemphigus foliaceus in Brazil, which concentrates in specific geographic areas. As the distance increases from these regions, the disease becomes less common. Certain drugs can produce an autoimmune response: procainamide (Pronestyl) commonly produces a lupuslike syndrome. Sometimes our own antigens can be altered; viruses, for example, can invade a cell and commandeer its genetic apparatus so that the immune system no longer recognizes the cell as self and begins to attack our own tissues. In other instances, antigens can have such similar components that an antibody manufactured to dispose of one reacts with another, even though they are not identical. (This is called molecular mimicry.) In this way an illness (like streptococcal infection) can provoke an immune response that continues to attack our own tissues after the infecting agent is long gone.

Scientists don't really understand precisely how the cells of our immune system learn to distinguish what is us from what is foreign and threatening. They have advanced a variety of theories to explain how it happens. One idea is that in the process of maturing, the cells that make up the immune system are exposed to all of the potential target molecules in the body's tissues to which they might react (that is, our own antigens) and, while still in an early stage of development, are signaled by what scientists call suppressor circuits not to turn on and mount a defense against the antigens of our own tissues. Those T cells that don't "learn" to ignore the body's own antigens may be programmed for death while they are maturing in the thymus, a process known as negative selection. In this way, amnesty for self is permanently built into our immune system and allows us to escape attack.

Another theory suggests that our immune cells "see" all target molecules, whether they are on the cells of our own tissue or are associated with foreign entities like bacteria. But before they turn on to attack any of those molecules, they must have a signal from a cooperating or helper cell. The helper cell does not provide that signal if the molecule is part of our own tissue. A third theory proposes that a whole network of groups of specialized cells are involved in preventing antibodies to our own tissues, even if we do make them, from ever reaching those tissues. The most current thinking is that since there is no essential difference between our own and foreign antigens, our protection depends on the fact that *lymphocytes evolved to respond to antigens only under certain circumstances,* generally in the presence of chemicals (cytokines) that produce inflammation in the tissue under attack.[1] This school of thought points out that the proper formation and maintenance of a competent population of T and B cells require a continuous exposure to the antigens of our own tissues and that we all have a low level of autoreactivity that never becomes intense enough to be harmful.

Whatever the mechanism, the properly functioning immune system preserves the fine-tuned ability to let what is us pass without challenge, and it turns on only what is truly harmful to us. But any change in the complex balance and function of the hundreds of processes that keep us safe in a hostile world—even a change in the proteins that make up our own tissues and organs—can turn a protective system into one that attacks our own bodies. Women are significantly more likely to have this happen than are men.

Why Do Women Get More Autoimmune Diseases?

One of the most important features of autoimmune disease is that after puberty and during the childbearing years (and to a lesser extent even after menopause), it occurs much more frequently in women than in men. Moreover, during pregnancy, some autoimmune diseases improve (multiple sclerosis* and rheumatoid arthritis, for example), while others, like lupus, worsen. Once the baby is delivered, an autoimmune disease that seemed to sleep during pregnancy can reawaken with a vengeance, sometimes worse than before. Are hormones the trigger for autoimmune disease?

Some facts support this idea: hormones certainly influence the occurrence and the course of autoimmune disease. Many women report that the symptoms of their autoimmune disorders are worse during specific times of their menstrual cycle, and even in healthy women the amount of different cytokines (a chemical produced by T4 cells to fight off invaders) changes during each cycle. The symptoms of rheumatoid arthritis and multiple sclerosis are often both worse at the beginning of the menstrual period. Oral contraceptives are protective against these two illnesses, but they do not protect against lupus.

Several aspects of the immune system differ as a function of sex. To point out just a few: in women, antibody responses to infection are more intense; women are more successful in fighting infections than are men. They also are less likely to reject grafts of tissue or transplanted organs. Women have more CD4 T cells than men. Men and women produce

---

* Multiple sclerosis is a chronic inflammatory disease of the central nervous system.

different amounts of cytokines and chemokines; in laboratory experiments gonadal hormones help to regulate these levels.

I have already mentioned that the two subsets of T4 cells do different things. T_H1 lymphocytes make cytokines, which increase the inflammatory component of defense against invaders; these cells dominate the immune response in diseases like rheumatoid arthritis and multiple sclerosis. T_H2 cells, on the other hand, assist in the production of antibodies; the activity of these cells is greater during pregnancy* and in patients with lupus.

Estrogen itself increases the effectiveness of T4 cells, particularly with regard to their collaboration in helping B cells to make antibodies. It also increases the number of circulating T8 cells. Many researchers have emphasized the importance of the gonadal hormones (estrogen, progesterone, and testosterone) in the regulation of the immune system and implicate them as a fundamentally important factor in causing autoimmune diseases. One of the most active proponents of a major (if not exclusive) role for hormones (particularly estrogen) in intensifying the severity and frequency of autoimmune disease in women is Robert Lahita, professor of medicine at New York Medical College.[2] He points out that lupus, for example, seems to be estrogen-driven; it affects women ten times as frequently as men. Moreover, women who have the illness also have, in their bodies, an intensely estrogenic environment. Their metabolism of estrogen tends to produce very feminizing compounds, and they have very reduced levels of androgens: they destroy testosterone very rapidly. Interestingly, some men with lupus have higher estrogen and lower testosterone levels than healthy men.[3] The profoundly important role of estrogen in lupus is further emphasized by the fact that with menopause lupus becomes less severe, but with pregnancy it worsens. For this reason, doctors are experimenting with using dihydroepiandrosterone (DHEA), a weakly androgenic hormone that dampens the T_H2 response (which fosters the production of antibodies), in treating women with lupus.

---

* This is the reason pregnancy dampens the activity of rheumatoid arthritis and multiple sclerosis: a T_H2 environment prevails, and the activity of T_H1 cells is diminished.

The sometimes apparently contradictory role of estrogen in modulating the intensity of autoimmune disease may be caused by the fact that, like all steroid hormones, its action is different at high and low concentrations. Estrogen, for example, enhances the activity of immune cells at low doses, but at high doses it inhibits them.

Autoimmune disease might be the consequence, among other things, of the failure of activated T cells to die after conquering the invader, which, in a well-regulated immune response, they do. If they do not, they continue to promote antibody production, and an autoimmune disease is often the result. Research in animals has shown that some activated T cells (generally T_H2 cells) persist longer in an estrogen-rich environment; others (usually T_H1 cells) survive better when testosterone is available. If the same thing happens in humans, autoimmunity based on the production of autoantibodies should predominate in females; autoimmunity based on cellular-mediated immunity should be more common in males.

Another factor implicating sex hormones in autoimmune disease is the difference in the severity of some of them in men and women. Although multiple sclerosis generally begins at a younger age in women, it is more severe when it does finally occur in men. Lupus starts during the premenopausal years in women, while in men it occurs much later in life.

Other experts in the genesis of autoimmune diseases don't think the answer is as simple as whether the patient is producing predominantly estrogen or testosterone. One of the most original and creative thinkers about the role of gender in the autoimmune process is Michael Lockshin, professor of medicine at Cornell University College of Medicine, who says, "A common belief is that gonadal hormones explain why autoimmune illnesses mostly afflict women. I call [this] the hormone hypothesis. The hormone hypothesis may be wrong ... autoimmune illness is not a single entity, rheumatic illness consists of more than autoantibodies and the effects of hormones are too complex to yield so simple an explanation. Gonadal hormones may *modulate* autoimmune illness. *Causation,* and therefore sex ratio, is a different issue."[4]

Lockshin points out that if hormones alone dictated whether people developed autoimmune disease, women would have more severe disease than men but not more frequent disease. He suggests instead several very interesting hypotheses, all of which involve the assumption that environmental and/or genetic factors may contribute to women's susceptibility to autoimmune disease. One of his ideas is that autoimmune disease can be due to a defect in the way women's sex chromosomes develop.

Another process called imprinting may be involved in autoimmunity. Imprinting (inactivating one of a pair of genes) is important for normal development. As a sperm fertilizes an egg or ovum, the genetic material of both parents unites to form a series of forty-six chromosomal pairs, each of which contains a matched set of genes, one from the mother and the other from the father. One chromosomal pair, the XX (female) or XY (male), determines the sex of the child. In the case of some genes, one of them must become inactivated in the process known as imprinting if the finished individual is to be normal. This is also true of the sex chromosomes: women who develop normally have to inactivate one of their X chromosomes; this process is called *lyonization*. In some of their cells, the paternal X may be inactivated; in others, the maternal X. Some of the genes on the inactivated X chromosome, though, don't participate in the inactivation process, which is under the control of a special gene called the X-inactive specific transcript (XIST) gene. If this gene is defective, proper X-inactivation fails, which can result in *sex-linked* diseases. Lockshin suggests that the gene that controls autoimmunity may be located in the X chromosome and be inappropriately inactivated, causing a predominance of autoimmune disease in women. It is well known that the X chromosome contains many genes responsible for coding the function of the immune system.

Lockshin points out some other interesting facts that indicate hormones cannot be the whole story behind autoimmune disease. People with diseases of the endocrine system (and therefore an imbalance in their hormonal milieu), for example, don't have an increased incidence of autoimmune disease. Furthermore, women given oral contraceptives or postmenopausal HRT don't reliably increase either the incidence or the intensity of every autoimmune disease. (In fact, several studies have suggested that they *reduce* the symptoms of rheumatoid arthritis and multiple sclerosis.) Finally, he says, if hormones are the sole cause of autoimmune disease, why does pregnancy neutralize the impact of rheumatoid arthritis and multiple sclerosis but intensify lupus?

Other hypotheses have been proposed to explain diseases that involve disruption of normal immune function. For example, in what is called microchimerism,* cells from two different individuals coexist in the same body, very much like a transplanted organ in a host. Interestingly, from the earliest stages of pregnancy, fetal cells can enter the mother's bloodstream and persist in the mother for as long as twenty-seven years after delivery. J. Lee Nelson of the Fred Hutchinson Cancer Research Center in Seattle believes that microchimerism lies at the basis of some diseases that are called autoimmune but would better be termed alloimmune; that is, diseases that are the result of the impact on immune function of cells that are of our species but not our own as individuals. Scleroderma is one of these. Nelson points out that scleroderma (also called progressive systemic sclerosis) resembles what happens to a patient whose body rejects a graft or a transplanted organ. This theory is supported by Nelson's work on a group of eleven women with scleroderma: nine of them had sons, and one of the others had had an abortion (the sex of that fetus was not known); in the last woman no history about previous pregnancies was available.

Chimerism may be operative in other situations. One thirteen-year-old boy with lupus had received an exchange transfusion when he was born. Maternal cells can enter the bloodstream of a baby during pregnancy; the child then has microchimerism. This is a possible basis for some of the (allo)immune diseases of childhood like juvenile dermatomyositis.

Work by other scientists supports the idea that hormones are not the whole reason for differences in the ability of males and females to resist an immune challenge. Cells isolated from the brains, hearts, and livers of embryonic mice so young that it was unlikely that their development

---

* In Greek mythology a chimera was a being composed of body parts of several different animals: the most familiar is the sphinx, with the hindquarters of a lion and the chest and head of a woman. The combination of cells of two different origins (fetal and maternal) is called a *microchimerism* for this reason.

was influenced by hormones had different sensitivities to lethal agents as a function of sex. Female cells of all three types were less able to resist the challenges and survive than male cells. The heart cells of both sexes were more vulnerable than those of the brain or liver.[5]

Researchers continue to be challenged—and puzzled—about why most autoimmune disease occurs more frequently in women than in men and about why the severity of those diseases can vary as a function of gender. Lockshin thinks we should investigate several intriguing possibilities. Among them:

- Defects in gene processing during development
- The role of nongonadal hormones like thyroid hormone and prolactin in provoking autoimmune diseases. Prolactin is particularly interesting because it promotes normal immune activity. (The severity of several autoimmune diseases can be mitigated by using bromcriptine, which suppresses prolactin production.)
- Sex-specific exposures to inciting agents (like the fetal cells that enter the maternal circulation during pregnancy)
- The possibility that normal sex-specific variations in human function may lay the groundwork for autoimmune disease. For example, late in pregnancy the ligaments that connect joints in women loosen, which could increase women's tendency to develop inflammation in those joints over time.
- The impact of sex-specific variations in anatomy and function, particularly that of the brain, on susceptibility to autoimmune disease
- Differences between the biological clocks (or circadian rhythms) of men and women. These can be important if cycling of hormones rather than the hormones themselves is important in promoting autoimmune phenomena.
- Whether a susceptibility gene is linked to an X or a Y chromosome. (This may be an important feature of how the severity of disease varies as a function of gender.)
- Cultural causes of sex skew of disease. (Women in some cultures eat the brains of the dead; kuru, a disease of the brain, is more common in such women; cultural factors can also influence hormonal levels

through environmental factors like stress: women's hormone levels may be differently affected by stress than those of men.)

Another intriguing notion is the idea that just as sex hormones influence the development of the brain (which is different in men and women), they may also influence the development—and function—of the thymus, which is very important in the maturation of the T cell and which is required to "instruct" the developing T cell about what is self and nonself.

While scientists understand a great deal about the immune system, their grasp of the reasons for the predominance of at least some autoimmune diseases in women is really inadequate. Recently, the proceedings of a conference on "Gender, Biology and Human Disease" were published, and in the paper summarizing the data that were presented, the following remarks appeared: "Most physicians believe that gender affects autoimmune disease incidence and severity, but definitions of gender, incidence and severity are inexact. From fertilization through puberty gender is plastic, prevalence figures are as much hearsay as fact and social and environmental influences on illness occur."[6]

HOW MEN AND WOMEN FIGHT INFECTIONS

Infections have different consequences for men and women. While hormones don't explain all of the variations, they play an important part in the intensity of the defense a person mounts: in general, testosterone dampens the activity of the immune system, while estrogen has the opposite effect. Consequently, women's immune systems are more active than those of men, and for that reason some vaccines are more effective in women. Polio virus, for example, provokes a stronger response in females than in males.

Even though researchers have been able to identify general trends like these, exceptions are plentiful, and we still aren't able to reliably predict gender-specific reactions to infections. *Sepsis* is a situation in which a bacterium and/or its poison products are so abundant that they invade the bloodstream and cause the patient's blood pressure to fall.

He or she may die in what is called septic shock—when it becomes impossible to keep the blood pressure high enough to supply vitally important organs like the kidneys, heart, and brain with enough oxygen and nutrients to keep them functioning. In one study of more than 1,300 patients, sepsis proved to be fatal to women more often than to men. Here, it seems, the more vigorous responses of women may actually be harmful in the face of a significant infection: they may actually destroy their own tissue along with the enemy. We know that severe infection stimulates an *anti-inflammatory* response in the body that protects us from overkill of the defensive response. Some scientists believe that death from sepsis happens when the balance between the two is disturbed. Others raise a recurring question: How do we know what is the result of a cultural or social variable, and what is the result of biological causes? These scientists point out that the men in this study might have come to the hospital in a less advanced state of illness; the women might have had less access to health care because they more often lived alone and were economically less advantaged in general than the men.

Here's another example from a recent study. Women who developed pneumonia during a hospital stay were twice as likely as men to die. This did not seem to be due to a delay in initiating treatment, and very little in the clinical response to the infections differed between the sexes, except that the women seemed to have less fever and higher white blood cell counts (a measure of the intensity of the immune system's response to the infection) than did men. But men stayed in the hospital longer after the diagnosis of pneumonia was made, which might have been a factor in their better survival rates.

The most salient examples in the discussion of infection and gender differences are parasites and the HIV virus. Let's take a look at the pathologies of these infections and what we know about the ways they differ in men and women.

Parasitic Infestation

One of the most interesting and well-established differences in the way males and females of all species react to infection is in the response to parasites.[7] Clinicians used to attribute these differences largely to external factors such as differences in diet (in some societies, meat is reserved for males, for example, while women and girls get the less expensive—and less nourishing—fare), differences in work, and even social customs, which can be quite significant. As I mentioned in Chapter 1, women in Muslim societies, covered in clothing from head to foot, are less likely than men to get malaria, which is transmitted by mosquitoes. Here's another interesting example. In the tropical climates of developing countries, women are more likely to get trachoma, an eye disease that can lead to blindness. The parasite breeds in fresh water, and because women are constantly standing in streams to wash the family clothing, they suffer more than men from trachoma. Boys' infection rates begin to drop when they reach puberty and stop playing near their mothers in the water. The same vulnerability of females around water is true with another parasite, the schistosomes, which are carried by the snail and enter the skin. One kind of water-borne schistosomiasis has a particularly high infection rate in women; the parasite that causes it *(S. haematobium)* infects the bladder and in women can infest the genital tract, bladder, and rectum; it can even cause generalized pelvic disease.

But while social and cultural factors are certainly contributing factors, scientists are now beginning to look more closely at other reasons for the sometimes striking differences in the incidence and severity of parasitic infections between the sexes. Does the parasite prefer one gender above the other? Or is the defense system of one sex more competent against certain kinds of attackers than the others?

Veterinarians have known for decades about differences between males and females in infestation with parasites. Male mammals have a higher rate of parasite infestation than females, and for males the infection is more intense. Heartworm, for example, that common pet affliction, is more frequent in male dogs than in females. In some kinds of infestations, other forces seem to outweigh the cultural vulnerability of women. For example, in some populations, men have a higher incidence of schistosomiasis than women, although women may have a greater exposure. In these groups, women may be more successful in mounting a defense against these parasites. Why?

Hormones may play an important role in susceptibility. During mating season, when their testosterone levels are highest, male ducks have more frequent and intense infections than females. Many other species (such as alligators, roaches, frogs, mice, cattle, and birds) have higher infestation rates in males than in females. A fascinating idea is that males with high levels of testosterone divert energy to producing secondary sex characteristics that help with mating (like the rooster's comb, or the antlers of a buck) at the expense of their immune competence. The best males, who survive to reproduce, combine immune competence *and* handsome ornamentation that make them attractive to females!

Several hypotheses have been raised to explain the peculiar vulnerability of males to parasitic infestation. One is based on the fact that males are *heterogametic,* that is, they have one X and one Y chromosome. Any potentially damaging gene associated with the sex chromosome would not have the bolstering effect of a matched allele,* which females, with two X chromosomes, possess. Any sex-linked characteristic in females would necessarily appear in a matched set. This is a great idea, but it actually doesn't fit the facts. There are species where the *female,* not the male, is heterogametic, like the wood duck, and the male is *still* disproportionately affected by parasites.

Another theory postulates that stress explains the difference in male and female vulnerability to infestation. It's well established that stress stimulates the adrenal glands to secrete the hormone cortisol, which depresses the immune system at many levels. Under stress fewer antibodies are produced, natural killer cells are less aggressive, and cytokine production falls off, among other things. During breeding season, males have to secure and hold territory, battle other suitors, and perform elaborate courtship rituals—all of which might be stress producing and depress the immune system. Unfortunately, there's no easy way of separating out the effects of stress in these situations from the effects of increased testosterone secretion, which accompanies all of these mating-connected behaviors as well.

At least part of the answer seems pretty straightforward: testos-

---

* An *allele* is the corresponding gene on the matching chromosome of a pair.

terone depresses the immune system. It may also have a direct effect on parasites themselves, helping them to be more vigorous and virulent. Some parasites initiate reproduction in response to the onset of sexual maturity in their hosts, as demonstrated in an experiment on infested mice, in which the parasite grows larger and faster in testosterone-treated mice than in nontreated mice.

MALARIA

Malaria is a particularly common and dangerous parasitic infection, particularly in developing countries. Pregnant women have a special susceptibility to malaria. The effectiveness of a woman's immune system is dampened during pregnancy, principally as a result of increased progesterone concentrations so that the mother will not reject the fetus. But this double-edged sword makes a pregnant female less able to defend herself against the malarial parasite. Malaria is one of the most common causes of death of young women in developing countries, in part because the malarial parasite lives in (and destroys) red blood cells. Many women in developing countries are anemic, having low red blood cell counts, and so they have a particular vulnerability to the disease.

Fortunately, if a woman contracts malaria during pregnancy, the antibodies she makes will cross the placenta and defend the fetus; congenital malaria is rare. On the other hand, if she contracts the infection for the first time during pregnancy, she has no antibodies to protect either herself or her fetus, which makes stillbirths and low-birth-weight babies more likely. As if this weren't enough, the malarial parasite may have a special ability to bind to the placenta. Not only does this make the placenta a reservoir for continuing infection, it probably interferes with the transfer of nutrients to the baby, which further explains the low birth weights. The other factor in vulnerability, though, is depression of the mother's immune system during pregnancy and into the immediate postpartum period.[8] Pregnant women should avoid traveling to areas of the world in which malaria is endemic, particularly Western women who have not previously been exposed to the parasite.

HIV and AIDS

Perhaps because it was first described in a population of homosexual men, acquired immunodeficiency syndrome (AIDS), which is caused by the human immunodeficiency virus (HIV), was studied principally in men. Now women represent half of the affected population in the world, yet the model for their care and for the behavior of the virus is still largely based on these original studies. In fact, the presenting symptoms of HIV infection in women are quite different from those in men, a fact that may be costing women their lives as doctors fail to diagnose them promptly and correctly.

Persistent and severe urinary tract infections or pelvic inflammatory disease may be the first clue that a woman's immune system has been compromised by HIV, but these are also common symptoms of other sexually transmitted diseases, and physicians may not consider the possibility of HIV infection until late in the game. The death rate of men with AIDS is falling by 3 percent each year, while that of women is escalating; our ignorance of how infection differs between the sexes may be contributing to this terrible situation. In 1985 about 93 percent of AIDS patients in the United States were men, but today 23 percent of new cases are women. The Centers for Disease Control and Prevention in Atlanta report that there are 120,000 to 160,000 American females with AIDS. Worldwide almost half the people who have AIDS are women! In all cases, a disproportionate number of both men and women are black and Hispanic.

There are important differences in the way HIV infection establishes itself as a function of gender. The infection seems to be correlated directly with the *amount* of virus to which a person is exposed; women seem to need only about half as much as men need. To put it another way, if equal amounts of virus were given to a man and a woman, the risk of infection for the woman would be 1.6 times greater. This is a very important point, since current guidelines from the U.S. Public Health Service recommend initiating treatment for HIV infection at levels (at least 10,000 copies/mL of blood) that were established based on research conducted exclusively in men! The chances of contracting HIV differ depending on mode of infection: one in

300–1,000 for receptive anal intercourse and one in 500–1,000 for male-female sexual intercourse. These variations are most likely due to the physical and anatomical differences between these partners and the amount of challenge they present to an invading virus.

Another interesting variation between the sexes is that in men, the virus seems to be all of one type, while in women, a single patient has more of a diversity of viruses. (Viral diversity, or heterogeneity, is important because the AIDS virus, once it has found a host, tends to mutate and produce alternate strains of itself. This makes it a moving target of sorts and is one of the primary reasons it is so hard to treat.) The diversity does *not* seem to be due to infection by multiple partners. In a study done on patients in Kenya, the number of partners had no relationship to the diversity of the viral load in infected women.[9]

The diversity of the viral population in infected women does not seem to be the result of more mutation in the female host; it is evident immediately. Women's particular anatomy might be a factor: semen can survive for days in the vagina and may continue infecting the female for days after intercourse with a larger and more varied population of virus than is the case in males. It may be that women can't selectively "filter out" any of the inoculating viral agents (as men may be able to do), and that some variants are more lethal than others, possibly placing women at a spectacular disadvantage in their fight against the disease. A contradictory theory has it that the presence of more variants may widen the umbrella of the immune response and actually make the disease less rather than more virulent in the female. But we don't yet know what relationship the number of variants bears to the severity of disease.

Scant but intriguing data connect infection rates and the course of the disease with hormone levels in women. Some scientists think high levels of progesterone (which occur after ovulation) may be marginally helpful in combating the rate at which the virus replicates. (In a small, 14-patient study, viral load dropped significantly in midcycle in women who ovulated.)[10] Data also suggest that HRT may help postmenopausal women with AIDS survive longer. Clearly, further research in these areas is warranted.

STRESS AND THE IMMUNE SYSTEM

Our state of mind unquestionably has a direct relationship to how well we fight off illness. A study of 90 newlywed couples showed that marital conflict had a profound effect on immune function, particularly in women.[11] In both sexes, stress reduced the production of antibodies, and the activity of natural killer cells was depressed. Ongoing stress may have even longer-lasting repercussions. Both current and former caregivers for Alzheimer's patients showed depressed immune function compared with normal individuals; 70 percent of these caregivers were women.

Like stress, depression dampens immune function. Recently bereaved people show diminished responses to immune stimuli for an average of two months after their loss.

These data are important for defending against particular diseases. A positive attitude and optimal mental health seem to influence the course of illnesses that depend on a vigorous immune response. Cancer is one of these, because the immune defense is very important to preventing metastases (the spreading of tumors from the original location to other sites in the body). In women with breast cancer, depression is associated with shorter survival times, while a sense of well-being predicts longer lives. Anxiety in HIV positive men has been associated with a more rapid course of disease, and infections were more frequent in volunteers inoculated with cold virus who were stressed than in those who were not.

Social support seems to stave off depression as well as feelings of isolation and loneliness. It definitely helps to maintain better immune function. In a study of caregivers for Alzheimer's patients, those that had a good network of helpful and empathetic friends had an improved ability to mount a good response to hepatitis B inoculation as well as better resistance to infection. Possibly most interesting of all, patients with some involvement in religion survive longer than those who do not—most studies show a 25 percent reduction in the likelihood of dying for such people. When men infected with HIV were involved in regular religious activity, they had significantly higher CD4 T cell counts, less depression, and less anxiety.

WHAT DOES THE NEW SCIENCE MEAN FOR YOU?

———

Since I had a severe flulike illness about two years ago, I've had a mysterious group of symptoms that no one seems able to explain or to relieve. My joints and muscles ache periodically, I sometimes run a low-grade fever, and although I sleep for twelve or fourteen hours, I wake up not feeling rested at all. I am completely exhausted. My worst time of the day is always the same—six o'clock in the evening, lasting for about two hours. Hives are a prominent part of my problem: unless I take a long-acting antihistamine every day, the slightest friction on or stroke along my skin produces huge red itching wheals. I've seen many doctors, I've had literally dozens of tests, and no one seems able to help me. Most have suggested a psychiatrist because they believe I'm depressed. Of course I am, but only because this illness has been so debilitating. I've been unable to work and even have trouble concentrating. What is wrong with me?

We have a lot to learn about autoimmune diseases, and some of them remain enormously puzzling, even to the experts. You are probably suffering from one of them. The two best-known diseases of this type are fibromyalgia and chronic fatigue syndrome.

Your description is dominated by your report of intense, unremitting, and debilitating fatigue. Presuming doctors have ruled out another cause for your symptoms (such as the better-defined autoimmune disease lupus erythematosus, which can take years to develop and may present as extraordinary fatigue), you may have what the NIH has termed chronic fatigue syndrome.

Here are the criteria for the diagnosis of chronic fatigue syndrome, according to the NIH:

1. Thoroughly evaluated, unexplained, persistent, or relapsing chronic fatigue that is of new onset, is not the result of ongoing exertion, is not substantially alleviated by rest, and results in substantial reduction in previous levels of activities.

2. The accompanying occurrence of four or more of the following symptoms, all of which must have persisted or recurred during six or

more consecutive months of illness and must not have predated the fatigue:

- Self-reported impairment in short-term memory or concentration
- Sore throat
- Tender cervical or axillary lymph nodes
- Muscle pain
- Multijoint pain without joint swelling or redness
- Headaches of a new type, pattern, or severity
- Unrefreshing sleep
- Postexertional malaise (feeling exhausted, aching, and generally unwell after even minimal exercise) lasting more than twenty-four hours.

Although the cause of this illness is unknown (and it may in fact represent a whole constellation of related diseases), here's what we do know about it:

- It's probably not contagious, although occasionally people in the same family or close contacts become ill at about the same time.
- The typical patient is a Caucasian woman between her mid-twenties and late forties, although men and women of all ages, races, and socioeconomic groups have contracted it.
- The disease is not rare: there are at least four to ten cases per 100,000 adults eighteen years of age or over.

Here's what you can do about it:

- Consult the Web for reputable information resources. The best data come from websites maintained by the National Institute of Allergy and Infectious Diseases, which is responsible for funding and doing research in this area and for developing educational pieces for the lay and professional communities and the Centers for Disease Control and Prevention in Atlanta. Some of the best sources of information have these URLs: www.immunesupport .com and www.niaid.nih.gov.

- Find a competent and well-informed physician with whom you can pursue appropriate diagnostic testing, and try carefully thought-out treatment that may help alleviate your symptoms.
- Consider contacting or visiting centers of excellence for the diagnosis and treatment of the disease, like the International Center for Interdisciplinary Studies of Immunology at Georgetown University Medical Center. Recent research there has proven quite exciting. For example, Joseph Bellanti, founder and director of the center, has identified a urinary marker of the disease that is simple to test for. The levels of this chemical returned to the normal range in affected patients who were taking a new dietary supplement, Enada/NADH, which caused a fourfold improvement in chronic fatigue syndrome sufferers.

I'm thirty years old, and I've had a real problem lately with a gritty, itchy feeling in both eyes. The pharmacist advised artificial tears, which have certainly helped, but I wonder whether I should see a doctor, because the relief is only temporary.

Chronically dry eyes in younger women should be evaluated by a physician: they are often the first symptom of an autoimmune disease like lupus, Sjögren's disease, or even rheumatoid arthritis. It's especially important to see your doctor if your joints have been hurting too; simple tests can rule out the possibility of something more serious than dry eyes.

I recently went on a camping trip with my wife; we seem to have eaten the same food and done the same things, including bathing in some delightful freshwater streams. I came home with a persistent diarrhea and stomach cramps, but she seems fine. What could be different about us that protected her from the problem?

Although I'm not aware of any data in humans, your particular vulnerability may be that you have more testosterone than your wife! Veterinarians know that male animals have a much greater susceptibility than females to parasitic infections. One postulated reason is the well-known tendency of testosterone to depress the immune system. You should be tested for infestation with *Giardia lamblia,* which is notorious for infecting swimmers in infested waters; a course of the antibiotic Flagyl might cure your symptoms.

I'm thinking of taking my wife to Africa as an anniversary present; we're planning a safari and expecting to explore some really interesting geography. She's three months pregnant, though. Should we put the trip off until after the baby is born?

Check the areas you plan to visit very carefully with a physician who is a specialist in tropical diseases or travel-related medicine. Women have a special vulnerability to malaria when pregnant, because their immune system is less active during this time. If your wife were to contract the disease, a miscarriage would be a very real risk, because vulnerability to malaria is most pronounced in the second and third trimesters.

I have had a very bad time with repeated vaginal and urinary tract infections that don't yield easily to antibiotics and recur as soon as I stop taking medication. Can something else be going on?

As alarming as it may seem, you should ask your doctor for an HIV test: the presenting symptoms in women of HIV infection are quite different from those of men. Genitourinary tract infections of particular intensity are often the first signal of immunocompromise in women.

I'm going through a difficult separation from my husband; he will probably be initiating divorce proceedings in the very near future. Ever since he left, I've been plagued with one cold after another. Is this just a coincidence?

No. Women are more likely to experience severe stress as a result of a disturbance or loss in personal or family relationships than are men. Stress and depression both dampen immune function, and the result can be both increased frequency of illnesses and more severe symptoms than in other individuals.

CHAPTER 7

The Skeleton

~~~~~~~~~~~~~~~~~~~~~~~~~~~~~~~~~~~~~~~

I'T'S EASY TO envision the skeleton as a kind of framework on which body parts are arranged, like clothes on a dressmaker's dummy. In this stereotypic view, the skeleton is alive only while we're still growing, after which it becomes so inert and durable that it's all that remains of us after our bodies have withered and turned to dust. But our bones are more than just a rigid system of struts. The skeleton is a living tissue that serves as a source of the calcium we need as well as a surface to which our muscles attach in a mutually beneficial arrangement: bone gives muscle an anchor against which to pull, and the tug of active muscle on bone stimulates bone formation. Without regular stimulation from muscles, bones begin to lose their mass. Even brief bedrest leads to a loss of bone that can become devastating, even in the young.

WE MAKE ONLY ENOUGH BONE
TO MEET OUR NEEDS

The economy of bone has to be very precise. The mass of the skeleton must be just enough to bear our weight and support the tug of active muscles attached to it. If it is too dense, it will become a burden to maintain. We are so brilliantly designed that our skeletons monitor themselves daily to support the forces that actually impact us. When bone is not stimulated by activity, bone mass immediately decreases. If, on the other hand, you begin to support more weight or exert a stronger pull on your muscles, your skeleton responds by increasing its bulk. These critical levels, below which bone atrophies and above which it grows, are called *set points*. This is the reason weight-bearing exercise is so important for maintaining an adequate bone mass and to help protect you against fractures.

How is the tug of active muscle on bone translated into a signal that "turns on" the production of more bone? Scientists do not really know, but they theorize that a tiny deformity on a bone's surface at the point of muscle pull stimulates cells (called *osteoblasts*—literally, "bone-builders") there to send a message, through a system of tunnels (canaliculi), to cells deep within the bone called *osteocytes*. In response to the signal, osteocytes (which are actually osteoblasts that have become incorporated into the bone itself) lay down new bone. Another group of cells balance their activity by not letting bone mass get too large; these are the *osteoclasts* (literally, "bone-breakers"). A complex cross-talk takes place between bone-forming cells and bone-digesting cells. In what are called *bone-forming units*, the osteoclasts munch away at bone, leaving it pitted with holes (cavities). As they do so, they secrete chemicals that signal the osteoblasts to lay down new bone and fill the cavities with a collagen-rich material called matrix. Matrix is a kind of scaffolding for new bone on which minerals (including calcium, phosphorus, sodium, carbonate, and magnesium) are then put into place. Calcium and phosphorus are the most important of these minerals; we turn over about 500 mg of calcium each day.

Bone production and the resorption of minerals go on constantly, and their balance is what maintains our bone thickness (density) at optimal levels. But when bone destruction outpaces bone production, we lose bone, sometimes to levels that result in deadly fractures. Our ability to maintain the balance depends on a variety of things: specific genes, bone size, body shape, body weight, muscle strength, and physical activity. Importantly, hormones also affect bone composition, producing many gender-specific differences in bone production and loss. These hormones include not only the gonadal hormones but also *parathyroid hormone* (PTH), produced by one of the four parathyroid glands (which lie in the neck just under the thyroid gland). This hormone regulates the levels of calcium and phosphorous in the blood; when calcium levels fall, PTH draws the mineral out of the bone. This same hormone also signals the kidneys to make 1,25 dihydroxy vitamin D, which we need to absorb calcium from our intestine. (This is the official name of the molecule; 1 and 25 are the carbon atoms to which hydroxy groups are attached.)

Osteoblasts, the bone-builder cells, have gender-specific features. When scientists looked at the characteristics of this kind of cell in pre- and postmenopausal women and compared them to those of men of the same age, they found that the osteoblasts in women were more affected by aging. In postmenopausal women, the cells were not only less active; they were fewer in number than in men of the same age. This is one reason older women are at particular risk for dangerous thinning of the bones, the well-publicized disease called *osteoporosis*.

HOW MALES AND FEMALES BUILD GENDER-SPECIFIC SKELETONS

For both sexes, bones not only grow longer during adolescence; they increase in mass and change in shape. Before puberty bone growth takes place mainly in the legs, but after puberty most of the growth is in the trunk. Between puberty and young adult life, bone mass *doubles*. Hormones play a vital role in this and in all skeletal growth and development: the gonadal hormones—estrogen, progesterone, and testosterone—help maintain the balance between bone formation and bone loss. Osteoblasts and osteoclasts are both sensitive to these hormones. (Specific molecules in their interiors serve as receptors for estrogen and testosterone.) So our height and shape change dramatically during puberty, when the production of estrogen and testosterone surges. Growth hormone, which stimulates the production of a hormone called insulinlike growth factor 1, is another essential part of the process in both sexes.

Bones grow and take shape differently in boys and girls.[1] At puberty all children grow taller by forming new bone in areas of special tissue at the end of their bones called the *epiphyses,* or growth plates. As long as the epiphyses continue to form new bone, children grow taller. But boys have a different growth pattern from girls. In the first place, boys have two more years of prepubertal growth, because for them puberty comes two years later, at about age fourteen. Puberty ushers in a time of rapid growth that lasts about three years in girls, and four years in boys. A study of the changes in bone during puberty in 107 girls showed that in early puberty most of the increase in bone mass is due to an increase in bone *size,* while in late puberty the bone becomes more *dense.* If illness arrests a child's growth, the impact on the skeleton will be different depending on the child's age when the disease occurs.

In late puberty, in response to a signal from estrogen, the epiphyses close. This occurs in boys as well as in girls; boys convert testosterone into the necessary estrogen by means of an enzyme called *aromatase.* Some men, who either don't have aromatase or don't have receptors for estrogen in their bones, continue to grow and achieve enormous height! In a groundbreaking case, John Bilezikian of Columbia University College of Medicine treated such a patient who lacked aromatase with estrogen replacement—which closed the epiphyses, stopped the patient's growth, and improved his severe osteoporosis.[2] This is what is called a prismatic case: one patient's illness and how we cure it gives us a new insight into how something works (in this case, how bone growth stops).

During adolescence and young adulthood, we all have a unique opportunity to build bone mass against the future (a little like making deposits in a bone bank, on which we can draw as we age). The window of time for building bone, unfortunately, is quite limited: in the third decade of life (a little earlier in women than in men) a subtle and (so far) inevitable disturbance in the balance of bone formation and destruction begins, as bone loss starts to exceed bone formation. This age-related bone loss is more intense in women, particularly in their vertebrae. Bone mass in females is maximal and plateaus at about twenty, while that of men continues to increase until about age twenty-six. Females' vertebral bones are densest during adolescence but lose mass each decade thereafter.

Unfortunately, most people don't take full advantage of this once-in-a-lifetime opportunity to make deposits into their bone banks. Teenagers need 1,300 mg of calcium a day, according to recently revised guidelines from the National Academy of Sciences. But the *Journal of Adolescent Health* has published a 1996 study showing that *only an astonishing 2 percent of fifteen-to-eighteen-year-old American girls get the calcium they need!*

OSTEOPOROSIS

In midlife bone mass is relatively constant for both sexes, but at menopause women undergo a period of particularly rapid bone loss (called type 1 osteoporosis) due to a marked increase in bone resorption that is not balanced by increased bone production. The menopausal fall-off in estrogen levels is partly responsible for this bone loss but not entirely. Only 20 percent of women develop osteoporotic fractures within twenty years of stopping their menses, and these women do not always have more estrogen deficiency than other same-age women. Caffeine consumption, lack of exercise, certain genetic factors, and smoking all influence whether a woman will develop osteoporosis and bone fractures later in life.

We know now that age-related bone loss is not the same for everyone, but varies tremendously from person to person. Some of the variation in bone density between individuals is unquestionably due to differences in genetic composition. Recent research about the vitamin D receptor gene has shown, for example, that this gene has several variants in humans and that each one has a different impact on bone density, even in people of the same age. A study of prepubertal girls found that individuals of the same age responded quite differently to identical calcium loads: when their diets were supplemented with identical amounts of calcium, they built up different levels of bone mass, depending on their genotype. In young men, one variant of the gene seems to be associated with higher-than-normal levels of circulating parathyroid hormone (as I will discuss in greater detail shortly). One group of investigators concluded that differences in the vitamin D receptor genes affect women much more than men, who seemed to have no difference in bone mass or in number of vertebral fractures as a consequence of such variations.[3] (The men and women subjects had similar numbers of each of the three possible genotypes being studied, so it seems that the men were actually less sensitive and not simply less likely to have variations.) Another interesting conclusion of the study was that the differences in genetic makeup affected the amount of peak bone mass women developed during adolescence more than they affected the speed or extent of bone loss after menopause. Other researchers have found that differences in the genes responsible for the production of estrogen receptors are also relevant to bone density. Recognizing these differences can help doctors identify patients who are at risk for bone loss, much the way they can now identify patients with greater risk for heart disease and hypertension by examining their family's disease history.

A common perception has it that osteoporosis occurs only in the elderly or the bedridden. Unfortunately, it's not true. At least once a month I must send a young woman not yet twenty for a bone density test, because I suspect she has severe depletion of bone mass due to an eating disorder. More often than not, my fear is confirmed. A disturbing triad is particularly prevalent in young dancers and athletes: amenorrhea (loss of menstrual periods), eating disorders, and osteoporosis. Young men have eating disorders too: as we saw in Chapter 4, when sports (like gymnastics) call for low body weight, males are at as great a risk as females, particularly for bulimia, to keep their bulk down to competitive levels. Very little data on the bone mass of these young men exist, but we know that in young women, when the ovaries hibernate because of starvation from an eating disorder, estrogen levels fall to the extent that bone is in negative balance and its mass can become dangerously depleted. These girls (sometimes astonishingly young) have to be put on oral contraceptives before they pass the point of no return. If they begin to menstruate again, either because they are persuaded to eat enough to keep up with their bodies' demand for nourishment or because of the estrogen in the pill, they have at least a chance of preventing irreversible skeletal damage.

TREATMENT FOR OSTEOPOROSIS: IS ESTROGEN THE ONLY ANSWER?

Estrogen-replacement therapy conserves bone mass in postmenopausal women as well as in athletes who have stopped menstruating because of estrogen deficiency. Estrogen keeps the bone-devouring role of the osteoclasts in check; low levels of the hormone are associated with rising levels of tissue cytokines, which stimulate osteoclasts to multiply and become more active. Only a few years ago doctors prescribed estrogen with great enthusiasm for postmenopausal women to stop the rapid bone loss that occurs for about a decade after menstrual periods end. Estrogen undoubtedly does halt that process, but a study by Elizabeth Barrett-Connor, of the University of California at San Diego, and her colleagues, who have followed the health of a retirement community population for several years, produced a completely unexpected finding. In this population of postmenopausal women and men of the same age, Barrett-Connor found that estrogen levels bore no relationship to the number of vertebral fractures in women. But for the men, there *was* an association between total estrogen levels and the prevalence of fractures; the lower the estrogen levels, the more fractures existed—in the *male* population! Barrett-Connor wrote: "There is very little evidence that low levels of estradiol in postmenopausal women influence(s) bone metabolism. It is possible that only premenopausal estrogen levels, or levels greater than some threshold concentration, have an effect on bone."[4] In other words, while using estrogen *does* stem the rapid loss of bone in the immediate postmenopausal period, low levels of estrogen in later life don't have an impact on the number of vertebral fractures in women, but unexpectedly, estrogen levels in men *do* correlate with number of fractures. The reasons are still being explored.

Are other treatments available for women at risk for bone loss besides estrogen-replacement therapy? Absolutely. Very effective alternative therapies are available, particularly a new class of drugs called *bisphosphonates,* of which alendronate (Fosamax) and risedronate (Actonel) are examples. They increase bone mass and reduce the risk of fractures in porous bone. Bisphosphonate treatment should be supplemented by adequate intake of calcium: postmenopausal women need 1,500 mg of calcium daily, in addition to 400 I.U. of vitamin D to ensure adequate absorption of the mineral from the intestinal tract. Optimal exercise regimens should involve antigravity exertion like lifting light weights, but it's important to avoid stress on vulnerable mechanical sites like the knees and elbows. Running, for example, can do more harm than good.

Our dilemma with bone loss is that once it begins, it can only be slowed down, not permanently reversed. The improvements effected by HRT or by exercise programs are, at best, provisional solutions; as soon as either of these treatments is discontinued, bone loss resumes at exactly the same rate as before the intervention.

PARATHYROID HORMONE, GENDER, AND BONE DENSITY

The accelerated loss of bone in recently menopausal women gradually levels off and resembles that of men, who lose bone slowly with aging. This age-related loss of bone (which leads to type 2 osteoporosis) happens at about the same rate in both sexes and is influenced by a slow increase in the levels of parathyroid hormone. The purpose of PTH is to regulate the level of calcium in the body. Its role is complex and varies with age, menopausal state, and the bones on which it acts.

In the normal patient, PTH stimulates both osteoblasts and osteoclasts. But due to illness or age, PTH levels rise above the optimal levels, at which point the hormone primarily stimulates osteoclasts; bone loss is the result. PTH levels rise as we age probably because our kidneys are less able to make 1,25 dihydroxy vitamin D, which causes the intestines to absorb calcium less efficiently. When calcium levels fall, PTH levels rise. Increased osteoclastic activity releases calcium from bone, stimulating the kidneys to make more vitamin D and to conserve calcium instead of excreting it in the usual amounts. Interestingly, PTH pulls calcium from bone quite selectively. It protects vertebral bone and prefers to work on cortical bones, such as those in our arms and legs.* There may be a role, in fact, for using PTH to spare the vulnerable vertebrae of women with established osteoporosis, since in these women (most of whom are postmenopausal) levels of PTH are decreased and are more easily suppressed than in normal women. The parathyroid glands in these patients show a less vigorous response than normal to lowered calcium levels.

Normal PTH secretion by the parathyroid glands differs according to gender. Men and women have different circadian rhythms (twenty-four-hour patterns) of hormone secretion, and a different response to fasting: in women, the rise in circulating PTH is less pronounced and the kidneys conserve calcium less efficiently. These minor differences may have a cumulative effect in women over the course of a lifetime and explain their greater vulnerability to osteoporosis.

Primary hyperparathyroidism is a disease in which the parathyroid glands, for no apparent reason, secrete more PTH than normal. Until recently, routine blood tests for serum calcium levels on annual checkups showed that the disease is very common—and is three times more common in women than in men. (It usually appears within the first ten years after menopause.) Unfortunately Medicare's requirements for laboratory testing now mean that physicians can no longer order many tests that the regulatory authorities believe have no indication, and the test for serum calcium levels is one of them. Primary hyperparathyroidism is usually asymptomatic; not until osteoporosis is well established (often when a fracture occurs) can physicians discover that the problem exists, unless they are periodically monitoring calcium levels in their patients.

What makes one or more of the parathyroids begin to secrete more hormone than necessary? We don't know, but they do so more frequently in patients who have had radiation of the face, neck, and upper chest for acne (a common treatment in the 1930s and 1940s). Sometimes a tumor of the parathyroid, called an adenoma, is responsible and must be surgically removed.

---

* There are several kinds of bones, and each is individually regulated and shaped as the skeleton matures. The back bones, called vertebrae, are made up of *trabecular,* or *spongy* bone. The bone of the arms and legs is much denser and is called *cortical* bone. Hip bones are intermediate in composition.

How effectively individual people maintain bone mass is complex and varied, so physicians should follow bone density measurements closely (at least every two years) in susceptible patients and in patients receiving therapy to maintain or increase bone density. Many doctors tell patients, "You're okay, because you're on estrogen," and may even deny bone density tests to patients who are taking HRT because they believe such women cannot develop osteoporosis. But the story is far more complicated than that, and physicians should be sensitive to the fact that some individuals need combinations of interventions, including estrogen, bisphosphonates, weight-bearing exercise, and calcium/vitamin D supplementation.

Finally, medications like steroids can seriously deplete bone mass within a very short time, and patients who are on such medications, even briefly, should be monitored for changes in bone density and treated appropriately if it begins to occur. Often, for example, a patient is given a course of steroids that cannot be tapered as rapidly as usual; when the medication is reduced below a certain level, the symptoms recur and the patient has to stay on low doses of steroid for much longer than was originally intended. These individuals need closer surveillance for the impact of the medication on bone mass.

OSTEOPOROSIS IN MEN: A DIFFERENT DISEASE?

Osteoporosis is one disease in which the usual gender-bias scenario is reversed; we know much more about it in women than in men, on whom relatively few direct observations have been made. The situation for men exactly parallels that of women and coronary artery disease: women were thought to be virtually exempt from the disease, so most of the research on that illness was done on men. But women are not the only ones affected by type 2 osteoporosis: men suffer from it too, albeit less frequently. Lifetime risk for the disease in men has been estimated at 13 to 25 percent. (In contrast, the frequency of the disease in older women is one in two.)

As John Bilezikian points out in his overview of osteoporosis in men,[5] physicians don't know what standards to use to diagnose osteoporosis in men, since the research on critically low values for bone mass was done exclusively in women.[6] These values may not be valid for men, since men have larger bones and higher peak bone mass than women. Osteoporosis was thought to affect women almost exclusively, but now that we know this is far from the case, medical researchers have to develop new standards for diagnosis and treatment that will be effective for men!

The clinical picture for men is also a little different than that for women. In the first place, men do not experience the relatively abrupt loss of gonadal hormones that menopausal women do. Only if their testicles are removed will men show the rapid bone loss that is so characteristic of postmenopausal women. Men tend to develop osteoporosis in different kinds of bone, losing only a quarter of the bone density in the spine that women lose and a third of the bone density in the hip. Nevertheless, at least a quarter of aging men are osteoporotic (compared with more than half of aging women). The most important risk factors for men are smoking, poorly developed gonads, excessive intake of alcohol, and the presence of other diseases known to affect calcium or bone metabolism. Steroid use is an immediate and significant risk factor for bone loss in both sexes, and as soon as steroid therapy is begun, even for a short period of time, many physicians begin bone-replacement therapy with bisphosphonates, which lay down new bone and lessen the possibility of fracture. Other less common causes are gastrointestinal disease, hyperthyroidism (occurring either spontaneously or as the result of too much thyroid medication), anticonvulsant therapy, cancers that involve the bone, and high doses of chemotherapy for malignancies. In spite of the best research efforts, no clear-cut cause for osteoporosis in almost half of the men with the disease is evident.

Nevertheless, recent investigations have shown that *estrogen critically affects the aging skeleton in both sexes,* giving rise to the so-called unified hypothesis. In women, estrogen fall-off after menopause produces a unique period of accelerated bone loss that continues until compensatory measures call it to a halt; the rate of attrition then slows down until it precisely parallels that of aging men. And as I have said, while testosterone helps maintain bone, particularly in the arms and legs, estrogen levels are also very important for men. In fact, in four recent studies involving a total of 1,410 men ranging from young adults to the elderly, *estrogen* and not testosterone was the best predictor of bone mass at all sites except the long bones of the appendages.

In both men and women, estrogen has important effects outside the skeleton that are relevant to bone health: low levels at older ages result in decreased calcium absorption by the intestine, increased loss of calcium in the urine, and lower levels of PTH (by a direct effect on the parathyroid gland). The consequence is that so much calcium is lost from the body (in both sexes) that to keep blood levels constant, calcium is leached from the skeleton. Another reason for this bone loss is that estrogen's directly stimulatory effect on the osteoblasts is lost when levels of the hormone fall. (Men may compensate for this loss to some extent, because osteoblasts also have testosterone receptors.)

Studies on castrated male rats, as well as the descriptions of men who have been unable to convert testosterone to estrogen because of a lack of the enzyme aromatase, or who have a defect in the gene that produces estrogen receptors on cells, all show that estrogen, not testosterone, plays a central role in forming and maintaining bone mass in males.

Does this mean men should get estrogen therapy? Unfortunately, estrogen is feminizing, so doctors cannot give it to men unless scientists somehow modify that property. But when men (such as the patient John Bilezikian described) have no estrogen at all because of a lack of aromatase, estrogen therapy is beneficial and in small amounts does not affect male reproductive ability and other male characteristics.

Interestingly, osteoporosis in men is very much more frequent in patients with chronic lung disease. This illness is often treated with steroids, given either by mouth or as an inhaled spray. Steroids are known to cause bone loss almost immediately. A study on male war veterans with chronic lung disease showed that steroid treatment, whether by mouth or by inhalation, was an important factor in bone loss, and that even in some patients *not* treated with steroids, osteoporosis was more likely to occur than in steroid-treated patients.[7] Interestingly, this population of men had lower levels of estrogen than same-age men without the disease. Testosterone levels, on the other hand, were not different in the two groups.

SPORTS AND THE SKELETON

Knee Injuries

Unexpectedly, women athletes have been found to injure their knees much more often than do their male counterparts: the incidence is a spectacular two to eight times more frequent in females. In particular, women are very vulnerable to a tear in the *anterior cruciate ligament* (ACL), one of the ligaments that stabilize the knee: rupture of the ACL is two to eighteen times more frequent in females. This is a real issue for women in the military, as well as for women at all ages who play sports. The price women pay for ACL tears is not trivial: each injury costs about $17,000 to repair and requires months of rehabilitation.

The knee joint is the place where the two lower bones of the leg (the tibia and the fibula) connect with the femur, or thighbone. The interface is cushioned by cartilage and stabilized by a system of braces of tough connective tissue that, together with the great muscles of the thigh (the posterior hamstrings and the anterior quadriceps), keep the joint stable and all of its components intact when we twist, jump, pivot, or change direction while running. Alison P. Toth and Frank A. Cordasco at the Hospital for Special Surgery in New York have written an extremely useful review of the problem of ACL injuries in women, pointing out crucial differences in the skeletons, joints, ligaments, and muscles of the two sexes that predispose women to be particularly vulnerable to knee injury.[8] These differences include:

• Women have *wider pelvises,* with a more pronounced forward tilt. As a result, females tend to hyperextend (overstraighten) their knees as they attempt to land after a jump and keep their balance.

• Women's joints are more lax, in part because hormone levels (estrogen and *relaxin*) fluctuate during the menstrual cycle. Estrogen depresses the rate of collagen synthesis in tendons and ligaments, reducing their tensile strength. More injuries have been reported during the ovulatory phase of women's cycles, when estrogen levels surge.

Surprisingly, oral contraceptives (which it was hoped would eliminate this problem by keeping estrogen levels low and more constant) didn't help, possibly due to the fact that oral contraceptives increase relaxin levels. Relaxin, a hormone that is particularly abundant in pregnant women, is responsible for loosening the ligaments and tendons during delivery, so that the birth canal can enlarge and allow the fetus to descend. It's present in lower concentrations in nonpregnant women too, and its concentration fluctuates during the menstrual cycle, increasing during ovulation and afterward. Like estrogen, relaxin increases collagen turnover and weakens the tendons and ligaments that stabilize joints.

• *Muscle strength* is significantly different in the two sexes. To sta bilize their knees, women rely more on their quadriceps muscles than on their hamstrings, while men activate their hamstrings with three times the intensity of women when landing from a jump or changing direction while running. The hamstrings, moreover, are weaker than those of men. Frank Noyes, director of the Cincinnati Sports Medicine and Orthopedic Center, has commented that to prevent injury, hamstrings should be at least 60 to 70 percent as strong as the quadriceps, but in women the ratio is actually only 45 to 55 percent.

Another very frequent problem in young female athletes is *patellar-femoral dysfunction*, involving the patella, or kneecap. Particularly in the adolescent phase of rapid growth, the junction between the patella and the joint is unstable. The most frequent symptom is pain *behind* the knee. In some cases, pressing on the patella produces a sensation of crunching (crepitus). The problem is usually cured by doing exercises that strengthen the quadriceps (such as lifting a weight attached to the foot with the knee straight by flexing the hip).

Teenage boys, on the other hand, have a different problem. *Osgood-Schlatter's disease* causes pain in the front of the knee just below the patella, due to traction from the patellar tendon on the tibia (the larger of the two bones in the lower leg). As soon as the phase of adolescent rapid growth ends (and the growth plate or epiphysis of the tibia closes), the pain goes away.

Shoulder Injuries

The shoulder joint is formed by three bones: the collarbone or clavicle, the humerus or upper arm bone, and the scapula or shoulder blade. Four muscles help to stabilize the bone interfaces; together they make up the rotator cuff, which helps keep the arm in place against the shoulder blade. Many different ligaments (bands of fibrous tissue) bind the bones together in a stable arrangement. There are two common kinds of shoulder injuries: tears of the rotator cuff, and inflammation of the tendons that anchor the rotator cuff muscles to bone. Chronic rotator cuff tears are more common in men over forty, while tendinitis is more common in women, who complain of a deep ache in the shoulder and outer upper arm that limits arm motion out to the side or turning behind the back. (Many of my women patients with this problem have learned to hook their brassieres in the front of their bodies, because pain prevents their hand from reaching high enough to hook it in the back.)

Repetitive Strain Injuries

Repetitive strain injuries (RSIs) result from performing the same motion over and over during a particular activity, in a position that puts undue strain on a tendon, muscle, and/or joint. Many of these activities involve repetitive actions: computer use, playing a musical instrument, hammering nails, and even shaking hands over and over. All can cause an RSI. One of the paradoxes of computers is that they have made writing much easier and quicker, but because the typewriter provided a whole range of different actions in typing a single line (pushing the carriage back to write the next line, using Wite-Out for mistakes, installing paper, and more) that prevented an unbroken string of repetitions of the same activity, RSIs were much less frequent when people used the more primitive instrument.

Women are more susceptible to RSIs than men, at least in part because most office furniture is designed for men's larger bodies. Moreover, women still perform more "keyboarding" jobs than men. The two office positions most likely to produce an RSI are graphic artist and paralegal, both of which involve repetitive fine motions of the hands and fingers, often under pressing deadline constraints.

Some of the most important work in treating RSIs was developed by Emil Pascareli, who founded the Miller Health Care Institute for Performing Artists at the St. Luke's–Roosevelt Hospital Center in New York City specifically to retrain musicians of both sexes who suffered injuries from long hours of playing their instruments. Very soon his work extended to patients with RSIs from a whole constellation of occupations, and he developed one of the most important training programs in the country, teaching physicians and health care professionals how to correct maneuvers that were producing crippling disabilities. He would begin by videotaping the patient and then analyzing the tape, showing the motions and positions of all the parts of the body contributing to the injury. Often he modified the instruments themselves to eliminate special points of strain. One of my own patients at the Miller Institute was a teenage girl preparing for a career as a concert pianist. She had had no problem at all when her mother-teacher restricted her to Bach: the even emphasis and the precisely timed, regular notes of the music were completely innocuous, and she mastered them with no problem. But at one point she suddenly developed an almost paralyzing pain in her wrists, hands, forearms, shoulders, and back that impeded her progress. Her troubles began, it turned out, when she graduated from Bach to the romantic composer Brahms. This entirely different kind of music required her to reach for a much wider span of notes, to accelerate and decelerate the rates at which she played, and to constantly vary the impact with which she struck the keys. For the first time, she was also reaching with her right foot to depress and release the sostenuto pedal as she played. (This had never been necessary with Bach's music.) We showed her the tremendous difference in the way she had to use her body—particularly her head, neck, forearms, wrists, and fingers—to play the new kind of music and, within several months, retrained her so that her pain receded.

WHAT DOES THE NEW SCIENCE MEAN FOR YOU?

My husband, who's only forty-two, has been asthmatic for more than twenty years. Recently, he broke his hip while simply walking down the street. His doctor sent him for a bone density test, and we found out he has advanced osteoporosis. How could this have happened to a man?

Your husband has been using steroids as part of his treatment for asthma for over twenty years. Steroid therapy causes profound bone loss. Recently, doctors have begun to use the relatively new class of medicines, bisphosphonates, in patients on steroids, including men. Even if a patient needs only a short course of steroid therapy that lasts only weeks or a few months, he or she also needs preventive bisphosphonate therapy simultaneously.

I went to my doctor this week because of a nagging pain in the upper outer side of my left arm. She discovered I couldn't move my arm out to the side or put it behind my back without increasing the pain. When she said I probably had a rotator cuff problem, I couldn't believe it. I thought the rotator cuff was a shoulder *issue. When my husband tore his rotator cuff, he had to have a surgical procedure to correct it.*

Men and women tend to have different symptoms with rotator cuff problems. Men are more likely to have frank tears in the muscles and/or tendons that are involved in shoulder stabilization and movement, but women are more likely to have an *inflammation* of one of the muscle tendons. You've probably been asked to use a nonsteroidal anti-inflammatory medication (NSAID) like ibuprofen. Whenever women have an injury or infection, their immune system develops a more intense inflammatory response as a defense than does men's, so doctors rely heavily on using an NSAID as a first step in therapy for women. Hopefully, you won't need surgery. Putting an ice pack over the sore area for twenty minutes at a time several times a day will help, as will resting your arm in a sling—but *only for brief periods of time* so you don't lose muscle strength and range of motion. Your doctor also probably will prescribe certain exercises for you to do at home: one is to "walk" up a wall with your fingers to increase mobility of your shoulder joint. Another is to lean toward the affected side, let your arm hang at your side, and move it in a circle of ever-increasing size.

I have developed pain at the base of my thumb. What's causing it?

This complaint is peculiar to women and is due to osteoarthritis. In women, the articulating faces of the bones that make up the joint are of unequal size, and wear and tear of repeated motion can erode the cartilage and inflame the joint. Men almost never have pain in this particular location, because the bones that make up this joint are similar in size and shape.

What are the goals of a reasonable exercise program?

The goals are the same for both sexes: flexibility, strength, and endurance, but the starting points are often different for men and women.

- Flexibility is the total range of motion of a joint or group of joints. In general, throughout life *men have less flexibility in all their joints than do women.* In pregnancy, relaxin levels are increased and provide a significant increase in women's flexibility. Dance training impacts flexibility: professional dancers have unusually good flexibility of their ankles and legs (but no remarkable advantage in the flexibility of their upper torsos). Flexibility is also improved by increasing body temperature and doing resistance training. Age causes a loss of flexibility in both sexes, usually because of a loss of elasticity in the connective tissue elements that stabilize joints and attach muscle to bone.
- *Men have greater muscle mass and strength than women.* Women in particular have less upper body strength than men, so training exercises for women should be planned to concentrate on improving upper body strength.

My eight-year-old daughter is going to play soccer next year. What exercises will help her avoid knee injuries?

A conditioning regimen for girls and young women who are going to play sports that involve running, jumping, and fast directional changes should include the following:

- Start with *overall body stretching*, giving particular attention to the quadriceps and hamstring muscles.
- *Weight training* to increase hamstring and quadriceps muscle strength should be a focus of special attention by trainers and coaches.
- *Jump training* is important: one regimen, called *box jumping*, involves jumping from the floor to a sturdy box and back down again; boxes of various heights can be incorporated into individual routines.
- Exercises to improve *balance and coordination* are important; an excellent one is to practice walking on a lowered balance beam. Another is to stand on one leg, eyes open and then shut for as long as possible.

I'm a thirty-five-year-old woman trying to prevent bone loss in my old age. What's the best approach to take?

Be sure to get plenty of weight-bearing exercise; even walking is beneficial. Check your family history for osteoporosis; if your mother or other female relatives have had it, the odds may be greater for you. Make sure your diet contains at least 1,500 mg of calcium a day and that you don't smoke. Excessive dieting, even in the past and particularly if it was enough to stop your menstrual periods, is a virtual guarantee of osteoporosis in the future. You should have a bone density test as a baseline now, and if you require treatment such as a bisphosphonate medication, make sure your bone density is tested every two years thereafter.

CHAPTER 8

The Skin

$\backsim$

ASK A DOCTOR in a burn unit what he fears most for his patient, and he'll answer, "Infection and dehydration, both of which are likely to be fatal if enough skin has been destroyed." The skin is not simply an inert envelope packed with our tissue. It's actually the largest organ in the body—an immensely effective and diversified collection of specialized systems that, among other things, provide us with the first line of defense in a hostile world. (Among many other things, it encapsulates and contains the potentially deadly anthrax bacillus that we've recently heard so much about.) The skin also produces and anchors the hair, which protects us from the elements; together with the skin's rich system of capillaries and the sweat glands, hair is an essential modulator of body temperature. Skin keeps vital water from evaporating from our tissues and manufactures the nails that guard our vulnerable toes and fingertips, ensuring their sensitivity and responsiveness to stimuli so that we are able to explore and manipulate objects in the world around us. Finally, the skin even metabolizes drugs and hormones.

The skin has two layers, each of which has a very different composition. The thinner outer layer is called the *epidermis* or cutaneous barrier; underneath is the much thicker *dermis*. The epidermis is constantly being renewed. It's made up of tightly packed layers of cells called *keratinocytes*, which are produced in the lowest layers of the epidermis and migrate upward to the skin's surface, where they form the outermost layer (the stratum corneum). This outer layer of cells contains keratin, which is also found in hair and nails; this protein prevents the evaporation of water from the body and is gradually sloughed off by friction and pressure. Although the epidermis has the same thickness in both men and women, its development is slower in the male fetus than in the female because testosterone retards its development, while estrogen facilitates its maturation. This difference is thought to be one of the reasons premature baby boys are not as hardy as premature girls and are less likely to survive.

At the base of the epidermis are the melanocytes, cells that produce the dark pigment called melanin that gives the skin its pigmentation. Men have consistently darker skin than women because they have more melanocytes (and not because of hormones; it is true even in people who have had their testes or ovaries removed). Interestingly, when stimulated by the sun or pregnancy (a time of great hormonal change), melanocytes can produce more melanin, resulting in areas of darkened pigmentation, particularly on the face (melasma, or the "mask of pregnancy").

Under the epidermis, the much thicker dermis contains collagen (a structural protein that helps provide firmness and dimension to the skin), elastin (which gives the skin its elasticity and prevents it from wrinkling), hair follicles, sweat and oil (sebaceous) glands, blood vessels, nerve fibers, and lymph ducts. Under the dermis is an insulating layer of fat, which guards the body against extremes of temperature and helps give contour to tissues in sites like the face.

THE GENDER-SPECIFIC EFFECTS OF AGING AND SUN EXPOSURE ON THE SKIN

The frequently made observation that men age better than women, I have always thought, has to do almost exclusively with their skin—it's just different! Skin is thicker at all ages in men than in women, but skin thickness declines steadily throughout a man's life. Women, on the other hand, maintain a constant skin thickness until after menopause, when the skin takes a sudden hit. Declining estrogen levels mean the epidermis thins and isn't renewed as often; combined with the effects of the sun, this effect makes the skin leathery and tough. The dermis loses collagen and elastin, and the skin develops both fine wrinkles and deep furrows, particularly in the face, where the muscles of expression have produced a lifetime of smiles and frowns. Subcutaneous fat disappears, and the skin becomes more transparent, so that blood vessels and tendons become more visible and prominent. These changes, together with the brown spots of discoloration due to sun damage and smoking, betray the age of the patient, particularly on the backs of the hands, where skin atrophy is most marked. After menopause, healing is slower, infections are more frequent, and pressure sores are more likely to develop.

Women's skin has more estrogen receptors than that of men, and females require more estrogen to keep their skin moist, retain the fat layer under the skin, and prevent the loss of elasticity that results in wrinkling and sagging not only in the face but all over the body surface. One patient who was contemplating a face-lift laughingly told me she intended to ask her plastic surgeon to begin at her toes and pull all of her sagging skin and the tissues under it back into its original position! One of the benefits of HRT after menopause is thicker, more elastic, and moister skin. In fact, in rats whose ovaries were removed, wounds were quickly healed simply by rubbing estrogen on the injured surface. The hormone caused the production of a protein (transforming growth factor-beta) that is crucially important for healing. Apparently women who were prescribed estrogen cream to replenish an atrophied vaginal lining have tried applying the same cream directly to their face and swear it improves the complexion. (This is definitely what the Food and Drug Administration calls an "off label" use of a drug!)

One of the only benefits of gaining weight as women age is that it preserves a thick layer of subcutaneous fat that not only serves as a factory for estrogen compounds in the tissue but also helps maintain the moisture, thickness, and contour of skin. It's a consolation I point out to my patients who want to lose ten pounds (why it's never eight or twelve pounds, I've never understood) and can't manage to do it. Losing a great deal of weight, particularly postmenopausally, depletes the skin's subcutaneous layer of fat, so that the price a woman pays for a svelte figure is accelerated wrinkling. Skin has to be very elastic not to show the effects of rapid and dramatic weight loss, which it is usually not the case in older people.

There are two components to aging in the skin. Intrinsic aging happens independently in the skin, as it does in other organs, but the sun does damage from the time of a baby's first exposure to it throughout life and accelerates the formation of wrinkles and patches of discoloration. Perhaps counterintuitively, men are more sensitive to chronic sun exposure than women, and they develop more wrinkling than women who have been exposed to the same amount of solar radiation. Cigarette smoking also increases wrinkling, in direct proportion to the length of time and number of cigarettes smoked (measured as *pack-years:* the number of years times the number of packs of cigarettes smoked per day). One reason is that nicotine reduces the blood supply to the skin, as it does to all organs, because nicotine constricts blood vessels. Another reason is that smoking elevates carbon monoxide levels, which further depletes the supply of oxygen to the tissues. This effect is marginally worse in women: men's relative risk for wrinkling with smoking is increased 2.3 times over that of nonsmokers, compared with a 3.1 increase for women. Vanity can be a powerful motivator: dermatologists have found that women are more likely to stop smoking to prevent wrinkling than to prevent lung cancer! (For more on smoking, see Chapter 11.)

AUTOIMMUNE DISEASES AND THE SKIN

The skin is a powerful immune factory. As the first barrier that infecting agents have to conquer if they are going to successfully attack us, the skin is an important player in defending against autoimmune diseases.

The rash of *lupus erythematosus* gave the disease its name, because the concentrations of lesions over the nose and cheeks reminded the first observers of a wolf's mask: the name literally means "red wolf."

Estrogen increases the severity of lupus. It worsens in most patients during pregnancy, and the longer a postmenopausal woman uses HRT, the more increased her risk of developing lupus.

Scleroderma, another autoimmune disease, is four times as frequent in women than in men. While it affects many organs, it has a rather spectacular effect on the skin, which thickens and tightens to produce a characteristic appearance called "mauskopf" or "mouse head," in which the patient's lips are thin and pursed and the skin is drawn so tightly over the facial bones that the patient has no wrinkles at all. In fact, some women resist treatment because they like the incredibly smooth appearance of their faces!

The hallmark of *psoriasis* is red, flaky patches of skin due to the rapid production of new cells that never mature but are abundantly supplied with new blood vessels. Psoriasis affects both sexes equally, but women smokers seem to develop it more frequently than men smokers. In fact, particularly in women, smoking may precipitate the disorder. Women, moreover, are more likely than men to develop the sore, inflamed joints often associated with psoriasis.

HAIR AND HORMONES

Balding is as important an issue for women as for men. What causes it and how to treat it are some of the most challenging—and often gender-specific—issues patients and their doctors face. Hair loss can be temporary and innocuous, like that which follows the birth of a baby, or it can be profound, irreversible, and complete, involving not only the scalp but the eyebrows and eyelashes as well.

The skin produces hair in special indentations in its surface called *follicles*. At the base of this unit, *matrix* cells produce the proteins (called keratins) that make up the hair shaft, while melanocytes make the pigment that give hair its color. Hair follicles begin to develop at about the ninth week of intrauterine life, starting at the head and eventually covering the entire surface of the body except for the genitals, the palms, and the soles of the feet. Each of us has almost 5 million hairs.

Every hair follicle, as it develops, goes through three cycles. The first grows a hair (called an anagen), which then regresses into a catagen hair, which finally becomes a resting (telogen) hair, which is eventually shed. We lose about a hundred hairs a day from the scalp; individual hairs last about 4.5 years and grow about half an inch each month. Brunettes have the most scalp hair, about 155,000; blondes have 140,000, and redheads have only about 85,000.

Hormones have a profound impact on hair distribution and quality. Skin can change (metabolize) hormones into active compounds that modify hair's properties. For example, the hair follicle converts circulating testosterone into a more powerful version of the hormone dihydrotestosterone (DHT) through the action of the enzyme* 5-alpha reductase. DHT, a powerful androgen (masculine hormone), binds to a special DHT receptor in the hair follicle. Other follicles bind testosterone itself without converting it to DHT. These two versions of the hormone produce quite different effects: testosterone-sensitive follicles are located in the lower pubic triangle and axillae (armpits) of both sexes, while DHT-sensitive follicles produce the hair characteristic of men—beard, chest, upper pubic triangle, nostril, and ear hair. Some males called male pseudohermaphrodites are born without receptors for testosterone or DHT in their tissue. The alert doctor can diagnose them because they lack both axillary and pubic hair. When these children achieve puberty, like all males they secrete estrogen as well as testosterone from their testes. Since they are completely unable to respond to testosterone, they develop breasts and appear to be females, although they have the X and Y chromosomes that mark them as male.

Other males are born without any 5-alpha reductase. These children grow up with genitalia that are characteristic neither of boys nor of girls (ambiguous genitalia), but at puberty, when their testes begin to secrete testosterone, they develop clearly masculine genitalia and other characteristically male features, like a deep voice and a muscular body. They never develop male pattern baldness, though, and they have no hair in the upper pubic region. (Since they can't make DHT out of

---

* An enzyme is a chemical that changes the speed of a chemical reaction without itself being changed in the process.

testosterone the DHT-sensitive hair follicles that are located in these areas are never stimulated to grow.*) These conditions are relatively rare, but they do demonstrate the importance of hormones and genes on sex-specific characteristics.

The commonest kind of baldness in both sexes is the result of the action of testosterone; hence it is called *androgenetic alopecia*. The pattern of hair loss, though, is different in the two sexes, because the localization of DHT-producing and DHT-sensitive follicles on the heads of men is sex-specific, namely in the frontal area of the hairline and at the crown (the area covered by a skullcap). Some men have increased sensitivity or responsiveness to DHT. As testosterone in these men is converted to DHT, they lose the hair in the follicle, which is why in male pattern baldness the hair at the front of the hairline and at the back of the head near the top (vertex) is lost first. In the worst cases, only a fringe of hair (populated by DHT-insensitive hair) is left. Incidentally, male pattern baldness isn't a sign only of virility; the high testosterone levels and superabundance of receptors in the scalp for the hormone signal an increased risk for coronary artery disease as well.

Women, on the other hand, keep their hair at the frontal margin and tend to lose it uniformly over the rest of their scalp. The reason is that they have few DHT-sensitive follicles at the frontal hairline. They also have more aromatase, the enzyme that converts testosterone to estrogen, in their hair follicles and much lower levels of 5-alpha reductase than do men. If you observe the oldest women in a hairdressing salon, you can see the light reflected through their thinning hair off their balding scalps in a uniform way—except at the very front of the hairline, where it remains relatively abundant. Smart hairdressers have learned this, and in their elderly clients, they use frontal hair to cover the rest of the scalp and/or curl the remaining hair of the crown so that it covers more area.

Tumors of the ovaries or the adrenal glands cause women to pro-

---

* Unfortunately for these individuals, there are two types of 5-alpha reductase: type 1 stimulates oil production by the sebaceous glands in the skin, while type 2 is the form found only in hair follicles. These males lack only type 2, so that they still can—and often do—develop acne.

duce more androgen than is normal. In some cultures, women have normal levels of androgens but an increased sensitivity to testosterone or testosteronelike hormones. These women develop male pattern baldness, have hair in a masculine distribution (including beards and moustaches), and have acne.

Treatments for Baldness

New frontiers of investigation are opening up potentially promising treatments for baldness. Two sets of experiments have increased hair thickness in mice. The first, the result of work by Michael Detmar of Harvard Medical School's Massachusetts General Hospital, finds that a protein called *vascular endothelial growth factor* (VEGF) may have an important positive impact on hair growth. VEGF enlarges blood vessels in the hair follicle and increases the supply of nutrients to growing hair. Mice who were genetically altered to produce more VEGF than normal increased the volume of their hair by 70 percent![1] Columbia University's Angela Christiano, who herself suffered from an unusual kind of baldness, *alopecia aereata,* has traced the complicated genetic abnormalities that characterize families with this unusual illness, in which patches of hair loss either on the scalp (or, in the case of men, in the beard) come and go without any apparent cause. The basis for the hair loss may be an inappropriate attack by the immune system on the hair follicle itself. Researchers at the Howard Hughes Medical Center in Chicago have transformed ordinary skin cells in mice into hair follicles by introducing a protein, beta catenin, which substantially increases hair growth in mice. Unfortunately, *limiting* the number of scalp cells that are converted into hair follicles remains a problem, and this kind of intervention has a theoretical danger, at least, of making a kind of "hairy tumor."

SELF-INDUCED HAIR LOSS: TRICHOTILLOMANIA

Some individuals compulsively pull out their own hair, sometimes using it to stimulate another part of the body like the upper lip. The unfortunate malady known as *trichotillomania* can afflict people of all ages. In adult life, women are much more likely to have it than men, although in childhood boys and girls are equally affected. The intensity of the compulsion, not surprisingly, seems to vary directly with stress, but it also can increase when the sufferer's guard is down during periods of relaxation, like watching television or reading a book. People try to resist the impulse of hair-pulling, which leads to an increase of tension that is released as soon as they give in and tug the hair out. Any area of the body that has hair, not only the scalp, can be a target, and the activity can last for hours at a time. Treatment is usually a combination of an SSRI and psychotherapy, but the disease tends to be chronic and relapsing.

ACNE

In some areas of the body, oil-producing glands drain into nearby hair follicles; these modified follicles, called pilosebaceous units, cause acne. Androgens like testosterone stimulate these oil-producing glands. Anything that will antagonize, or slow, the production of testosterone helps control acne. Some birth control pills make acne worse because the progesterones in them are like androgens in their effect; the worst offenders are levonorgestrel and norethindrone. The newer birth control pills (desogestrel or norgestimate) are much less androgenic, and acne is not a side effect of these preparations. In fact, these pills (Ortho Tri Cyclen was the first one) are used to *treat* acne because they increase the amount of sex-hormone-binding globulins in the blood, which binds circulating testosterone and prevents it from stimulating sensitive pilosebaceous units.

SKIN CANCER

The sun, unfortunately, is not always our friend; we know this but don't always heed it. Whether we tan deliberately or simply live in sunny climates where sun exposure is inevitable, even the most cautious of us are likely to reap an unpleasant harvest of consequences, ranging from accelerated aging of the skin to cancers of the skin.

There are three common forms of skin cancer. *Melanoma,* the most deadly, is usually the result of extensive sun damage or exposure to ultraviolet radiation (the kind used in tanning beds to give you that deep, tropical glow).* The incidence of melanoma is on the rise (rates increased by 120 percent between 1973 and 1994), as are melanoma-related deaths. In 1998 a shocking *one in 80 Americans had the disease!*[2] All told, melanoma accounts for *six out of seven skin cancer deaths.*

Women's clothing generally exposes more skin than men's, which means that the distribution of these cancers in men and women is quite different. Men, who begin to have higher rates of melanoma than women after age forty-five, are affected more on the neck and ears. Women, on the other hand, have more *melanomata* (cancerous lesions) than men before the age of forty, and they tend to get them more frequently on the legs and hips (a penalty for wearing bikinis and skirts rather than trunks and long pants). For reasons not entirely clear, women survive the cancer better than men. In spite of the fact that some melanomata have estrogen receptors, neither pregnancy nor the use of supplemental estrogen in oral contraceptives or in HRT after menopause seems to worsen outcome for women with the disease.

The two other common kinds of skin cancer are *basal cell carcinoma* and *squamous cell carcinoma.* Both come from the keratinocytes in the epidermis. Squamous cell carcinoma is more likely to spread, but basal cell cancers are four times more common and can be very disfiguring. Unfortunately, both are becoming much more common and are more frequent in men. They are caused by sun exposure, for the most part. (If we could only convince our tanning-mad teenagers that they will pay later for those gorgeous brown skins they cultivate all summer long, we might really be able to put the brakes on this epidemic!) For reasons unknown, basal cells are twice as frequent in men as in women, and the ratio is even higher for squamous cell cancers. Again, the distribution of these cancers is sex-specific: they occur more frequently on

---

* Both kinds of ultraviolet radiation, A and B, are harmful to the skin. Sunblock protects only against A.

the ears of men and on the legs of women probably due to the shorter hairstyles of men and the exposed legs of women, since they are almost always caused by exposure to the sun. Interestingly, immunosuppressive therapy leads to a tremendous increase in the occurrence of squamous cell cancers.

I spoke to a patient recently whose entire nose and upper lip were eaten away by his basal cell carcinoma. Why had he waited so long to see a doctor? I asked. "I thought it would go away," he answered. It is very wise to have an experienced dermatologist check your total body every year: I have seen melanoma on the vulva, between the toes, and in the hair. One particularly careful physician I know looks at the scalp with a hair dryer, which spread the hairs evenly all over the head, so that he can see the underlying skin well enough to detect a lesion. Make sure your doctor looks between your toes, at your genitals, and on the soles of your feet, as well as at your scalp.

WHAT DOES THE NEW SCIENCE MEAN FOR YOU?

I'm a weight lifter who's used anabolic steroids to help build up my muscle mass. Recently, I've noticed I'm losing a lot of hair. Is there a connection?

Anabolic steroids, which are being used increasingly by young people, help increase muscle mass, but because they are parent compounds of testosterone, they have dangerous side effects, including diabetes, impotence, and high blood pressure. Another side effect is to increase hair loss in the sites most vulnerable to the impact of androgenic hormones. This can happen in female athletes who use steroids too: they can actually lose their menstrual periods and develop increased facial hair, male pattern baldness, deepened voices, and enlarged clitorises.

The extent to which young people use anabolic steroids shouldn't be underestimated. A study called Monitoring the Future has been conducted annually since 1975, surveying the habits of 45,173 young adolescents from 435 public and private schools in the eighth, tenth, and twelfth grades nationwide. In 1989 steroid use was added to the list of topics included in the survey. The data showed that most steroid users are male; in 1999, 2.2 percent of eighth graders, 2.8 percent of tenth graders, and 2.5 percent of twelfth graders were taking steroids to improve body muscle mass.[3]

I've been an avid sailor, tennis player, and snow skier for most of my life. Should I have a dermatologist monitor my skin for sun-related cancers?

Here are the risk factors for skin cancer:

- Light complexion. Light-skinned people are more than twenty times more likely to develop skin cancer than African Americans.
- Male gender. Men are twice as likely to have basal cell carcinomas than women and three times more likely to have squamous cell carcinomas.
- Previous history of skin cancer. Thirty-five to 50 percent of patients who've had one basal cell carcinoma will develop a new one within five years.
- History of chronic exposure to the sun, or severe sunburns early in life.
- Freckles, which are a sign of sun damage and sun sensitivity. If you are heavily freckled (or are becoming more so), you are likely to need sophisticated attention to your skin on a yearly basis.

If you have any of these risk factors, you should have a complete check at least annually by a dermatologist, more often if you notice unusual mole growth or changes. All kinds of advanced techniques now make it easier for dermatologists to catch cancers at an early stage. Some dermatologists even use special lighting and photography to examine and record the appearance of a patient's skin.

When I'm reading or watching a movie, I tend to twist my hair around my finger. Does this have any bad effects?

Twisting your hair around your finger does damage it and breaks off individual strands. The disorder is related to the more serious trichotillomania (pulling hair out of the skin), as are eating hair, pulling hair strands between the teeth, and even pulling hair from other people or pets! Nail biting and scratching normal skin are also associated disorders. All of these unusual habits have a much higher incidence in females than in males. If you experience this type of behavior, and it advances to the point where it is disruptive or painful, you should see a specialist who can decide how best to treat you.

Ever since menopause, my nails have developed longitudinal ridges that split the nail at the tips. What can I do about it?

HRT may or may not help this disturbing problem, which can be severe enough to cause bleeding and broken nails that cannot be induced to grow in aging women. Daily application of moisturizing cream at the base of the nail may be useful. Although dermatologists suggest avoiding nail polish, several layers of protective lacquer may ꞈꞈꞈ the nail to the point that it doesn't break off in the terminal part of the weakened ridge.

Although I am a woman, I have a noticeable moustache and coarse, dark chin hair. This is a new development. What should I do about it?

Most women with heavy facial hair have normal levels of circulating androgenic hormones; their facial hair is due to a genetic predisposition for a more-intense-than-usual response of the hair follicles to testosterone. If your facial hair has been a recent development, though, particularly if you are premenopausal, you should consult your physician to be sure you don't have a tumor of the adrenal gland or ovary, which could be producing androgenic hormones. Women with the functional disorder *polycystic ovary syndrome* (which is underdiagnosed) have a mild excess of androgenic hormones resulting in increased insulin resistance (which can be treated quite successfully with oral antidiabetic agents), increased facial hair, infertility, and hypertension.

My doctor put me on the pill, and I've developed acne again. I thought I was all through with this! What is causing it?

Ask your doctor to give you another kind of oral contraceptive, because the progestin in yours may be too androgenic. Some oral contraceptives (such as Ortho Tri-Cyclen, which is norgestimate/ethinyl estradiol) are actually useful in treating pre-existing acne.

My husband's baldness has responded well to a medication called finasteride. Can I try it?

Finasteride is not approved for use in women; it blocks the conversion of testosterone into dihydrotestosterone by inhibiting the enzyme that achieves this transformation, 5-alpha reductase. DHT is needed to masculinize the genitalia of a male fetus, so it can't be used by women of reproductive age.

One of the changes I've noticed since menopause is thinning and straightening of my pubic hair. Will estrogen replacement reverse these changes?

No; the quantity and characteristics of pubic hair are the result of testosterone, not estrogen. Your doctor may prescribe testosterone for some postmenopausal symptoms (see Chapter 10) but probably not for this one.

CHAPTER 9

Pain

NOTHING IN MEDICINE is so personal, so compelling, and so isolating as pain. The doctor can't measure it; frequently has had no personal experience of what the patient is trying to describe, and as a result, generally tends to underestimate and under- treat it. Because the most effective pain medications are addictive, the physician prefers to err on the side of caution when treating a patient, even when the sick person is dying. As for the patient herself, her inability to communicate the grinding constancy of often nearly unbearable pain compounds her plight with a terrible sense of isolation.

Doctors hate problems they can't solve. Rarely do we feel more helpless than when we can't put an end to—or even mitigate—a patient's pain; so we tend to minimize or even deny its existence. It's one of our worst failings. Excellent data support the fact that even a fetus can feel pain, and the assumption that a newborn baby boy can- not feel the pain of circumcision (or that, because he is tiny and with- out language, his pain must be diminutive as well) has now been utterly disproved.

Physicians seem to have particular prejudices about women in this area too. It is well established that women report more severe levels and more frequent and longer-lasting bouts of pain in more areas of the body than do men. All too often doctors assume that women simply are more willing to report pain's existence and to seek help for it; some researchers have lumped it in with what they call women's "health-seeking behavior" or have attributed it to a nineteenth-century view that some women still have of themselves as frail and unhealthy. In fact, new data from research done on female subjects suggests that the awareness and experience of pain, as well as the response to pain-relieving medications, does actually differ between men and women. This is one of the most interesting and potentially useful observations in the new science of gender-specific medicine.

On the first day of medical school, I have often thought, every student ought to have to answer the question, "What is the meaning of human suffering?" Since the daily business of doctors involves mitigating the pain and discomfort of their patients, both physical and emotional, all doctors ought to have an answer to the question. Mine has been refined considerably since my internship, when I entered the wards of Bellevue Hospital for the first time, thinking to myself, "Now I will really see suffering! These are the most destitute and abandoned people in New York City." Bellevue was a charity hospital, a patient's last stop when all the other hospitals were filled. When we ran out of beds in times of crisis, we brought up cots from the basement, and in the bleakest days of winter our corridors were filled with desperately sick patients whom our crowded wards could no longer contain. The first lesson I learned as a physician was that these poorest, most deprived people were no more happy or unhappy than my own friends and family. Pain knows no social or cultural barriers, and despair—or contentment—seems to depend on the inner structure of the person-ality much more than on the circumstances in which my patients find themselves. On those Bellevue wards, though, I did learn about pain. In that chaotic atmosphere, I learned about how human beings accom-modate loss and suffering, and how they metabolize even the bitter realization that they will not survive their illness. If suffering was too acute, I discovered, people simply succumbed. They died of it, or sank into despair. If a patient did survive, it often proved to be a remarkable stimulus for him to develop resources that he never would otherwise have had. Many died without protest, often quite courageously. Oth-ers, though, seemed constantly overwhelmed by much less serious threats, and some patients who were not critically ill simply could not be comforted.

The science of how animals, including humans, respond to painful (nociceptive) stimuli may help to explain the tremendous variability in how individuals perceive and react to pain. Doctors have been exploring this issue for many decades, albeit with sometimes primitive experiments. One physician reported in 1934 that a measured amount of pressure on the skull behind the ear produced marked pain in 60 to 70 percent of his patients, while the rest of them had little or no pain![1] Recent, more scientific studies have helped to explain these enormous differences between people. In the brain's response to a painful stimulus, many more areas of the brain are activated than we might have expected, and the number and location of these activated areas vary a great deal from person to person, implying that learned behavior (which would naturally vary from person to person) might play an important role, in ways we aren't even aware of, in our responses to pain. It also makes research in this difficult area even more complex. Finally, an important study about pain and the central nervous system has made the point that when we receive a noxious stimulus, areas of the brain associated with action are activated as though the brain were developing new resources to help cope with the challenge.

ARE WOMEN MORE SENSITIVE TO PAIN THAN MEN?

Some researchers believe there are real differences in how men and women experience pain based on their sex-specific anatomy and the function of some of the organs involved, most notably the brain and the peripheral nervous system. Others are convinced that any gender-specific variation in the experience and reporting of pain is overwhelmingly due to culture and conditioning and depends on the way men and women are taught to express themselves and the personal qualities they are encouraged to develop. (Boy toddlers who skin a knee are told to get up, stop crying, and keep walking; girls have their tears brushed away, get a comforting hug, and may even be allowed to get back into the stroller!)

Many factors mitigate the experience of pain and make real certainty about what is specifically the result of biological sex very difficult. For example,

• Women have different *strategies* to alleviate pain: they use more pain-relieving medicine and more adjunctive therapies like relaxation techniques, aromatherapy, massage, and visualization.

• In scientific experiments, when men and women are tested under controlled conditions with the same unpleasant stimulus, cultural conditioning seems to affect the results more than hardwiring. For men, but not women, the place the stimulus is delivered is important: men react more intensely if the lower abdomen near the genitals is stimulated. The gender and the attractiveness of the experimenter affects men's responses but not those of women: men report less pain when the observing scientist is female, while women show no difference when the investigator is male or female! The personal traits of the subject (level of anxiety, reliance on and development of personal control, and the like) also affect the data.

• Other biological issues that have nothing to do with gender confound the data. Nutritional status (particularly the intake of sugar and fat) and the presence of other diseases, for example, also influence a person's response to painful stimuli.

For whatever reasons, women tend to report pain with milder stimulation than men; they have a better ability to describe it, they tolerate it less well, and they feel it longer, more intensely, and in more areas of the body than do men. Some studies show that women experience more discomfort and pain from pressure and electrical stimulation than men, while thermal stimulation (heat or cold) and the pain that comes from cutting off the blood supply to a body part (ischemic pain) show fewer sex-specific differences in the response. But many of these experiments yield contradictory results, perhaps because they rarely take into account the fact that pain sensitivity in humans and even in animals varies with age, pregnancy, the menstrual cycle, and the use of exogenous hormones like oral contraceptives. Finally, there are sex-specific differences in the absorption and metabolism of pain-killing medications and anesthetics.

GENES AND PAIN

Some variability in the experience of pain is unquestionably genetic. Consider the remarkable story of the Human Pincushion, a carnival performer with a unique insensitivity to pain, although he could feel all other kinds of stimuli.[2] He had a defect in a specific gene, NTRK1 (not surprisingly called the Congenital Insensitivity to Pain gene). At least three different kinds of mutation in that same gene have now been identified, which produce a variety of defects:

- Over 40 people have now been studied who lack a specific receptor in their nervous system that makes them unable to complete the circuits necessary for registering pain.
- One hundred and two people from four related Australian families have a defect in the nerve fibers that receive sensations from the outside world (sensory fibers). All incoming messages in the affected people are muted, especially those that have to do with pain.
- Two sisters have been described who had a unique combination of a spontaneous and unprovoked loss of their fingers and toes and an inability to feel pain.

The defect in NTRK1 affects both men and women, but some of the genetic defects that result in pain modification are sex-specific:

- A male-specific mutation on chromosome 4 affects the time it takes for a rat to withdraw its tail after being placed on a hot plate; depending on the presence of the mutation, the time the animal tolerates the high temperature before removing his tail varies significantly.
- When mice are forced to swim for long periods of time, the brains of both males and females produce an anesthetizing chemical that

helps them tolerate the ordeal. This phenomenon is called *stress-induced analgesia* (SIA). The chemical comes in two different general types: one is called nonopioid, because it is not like morphine (it is not neutralized by naloxone, which is an antagonist of morphine), and the other is opioid (because it *is* neutralized by naloxone). Nonopioid SIA is different in the two sexes, a pattern set early in development. Male mice mount a more robust nonopioid SIA than female mice. The female-specific system has a different hormonal basis: it is dependent on the mouse fetus *not* being exposed to testosterone during intrauterine development; it emerges only after puberty; it varies with reproductive status; and it persists after the equivalent of menopause. Genetic analysis showed that the gene controlling SIA in the female mouse (but not in the male) is probably located on a specific site on chromosome 8. Variations in the gene are related to the amount of nonopioid SIA that different female mice produce; some produce none at all. All this is to say that, judging from their levels of these chemicals, the experience of pain in these mice may be more intense in the females than in the males.

• Other experiments in rodents have revealed an interesting link between the ability to tolerate pain and sensitivity to morphine. In general, when sex differences exist, it is males who show a significantly greater ability to tolerate a painful stimulus. These same animals also show greater responsiveness to analgesia: morphine has a greater impact on relieving pain in these "doubly advantaged" males.

• Pain-killing drugs have several kinds of receptors in the human brain. The two best known are called the μ-opioid receptor and the kappa or k-opioid receptor. Morphine, for example, reacts with μ-opioid receptors. In human studies, women seem more responsive to agents that interact with the k-opioid receptor than men: after oral surgery, pentazocine (Talwin), nalbuphine hydrochloride (Nubain), and butorphanol tartrate (Stadol) all worked better at relieving pain in women than in men. The superiority of these medicines in women was not influenced by the menstrual cycle (which means that hormones had nothing to do with the gender differences in response to these medications).

Genes affect the experience of pain in other ways. Some painful diseases only occur in one sex: only men get hemophilia, for example. Our bodies often process and use many drugs, including drugs that relieve pain, in sex-specific ways, which are importantly influenced by gonadal (sex) hormones.

DRUGS AND PAIN

The ways in which the body processes analgesic drugs and anesthetic agents affect how men and women respond to pain treatment. Differences in body composition can be a factor: men have more muscle mass and women more fat, but some drugs bind to fat cells, so the amount of body fat affects the duration of a drug's action. Because a woman's digestive system moves solids and liquids along more slowly than a man's, moreover, any pain-killer she takes by mouth may have a more potent effect, since it has more time to be absorbed during its passage through the digestive tract. The rate at which we process drugs in our liver and the efficiency and speed with which our kidneys operate to clear medicines from our system also influence the impact of pain-relieving medication. How people metabolize drugs as a result of genetic inheritance can also be very important: for example, 7 to 10 percent of Caucasians can't convert codeine to morphine because of a variation in the cytochrome P450 system in their nerves. Since the pain-relieving action of codeine depends on its conversion in the body to morphine, these patients get no pain relief from taking the drug— although they are still able to suffer its side effects!

ANATOMICAL DIFFERENCES
IN THE NERVOUS SYSTEM

Anatomical differences in the nervous systems of men and women may account for some important differences in pain perception. One sex may simply have more nerve fibers than the other in an area of tissue that receives a painful or unpleasant stimulus. Special nerve fibers, called *C fibers,* are activated by injury or illness; the impulses that result can produce changes that persist long after the stimulus is over. These fibers are abundant in the pelvic organs of women. As a result of vaginal and uterine vulnerability to painful consequences of intercourse, the birth of children, and menstrual cramps, scientists theorize, women are more likely to suffer pelvic trauma than are men. The C fibers "remember" these stimuli and not only produce a heightened awareness of pain in the affected organ they supply but carry impulses to other nerves in their travels up the spinal cord. This is thought to be the reason women experience more *referred pain* (pain felt in a place other than where it originated) than men, particularly in the muscles of the head and neck.

HORMONES AND PAIN

Hormones are key modulators of the experience of pain. They modify our ability to keep nerves in optimal working condition, and they regulate the production of nerve growth factor and a substance involved in our awareness of pain called P substance. Estrogen influences the size of the "field" of nerves that are activated in response to a painful stimulus. Estrogen binds to opioid receptors in the brain. Thus the number of receptors and their affinity for medications that reduce pain vary with the phase of the menstrual cycle. Progesterone desensitizes opioid receptors in the brain and produces hypersensitivity to thermal stimuli, as well as (in rats) diminishing the power of morphine to relieve pain. These phenomena help to explain why sensitivity to pain varies with the menstrual cycle; menstruating women (who have relatively less available estrogen) are often more sensitive to pain than at other times in the month.

The same areas of the brain that scientists have identified as important to reproductive behavior are also very important to the experience of pain, which may explain the apparent link between hormonal fluctuations and response to noxious stimuli. In fact, if a woman experiences pain at a time when certain hormones are more abundant, she may become permanently sensitized to the experience of pain and have hypersensitivity and/or develop chronic pain at the site of the original stimulus *even after that stimulus is no longer present*—much like the effect of C fibers, mentioned earlier. This phenomenon is evident in some patients after mastectomy. Instead of recovering uneventfully, about one in ten develops chronic pain in the underarm, the chest, and occasionally the shoulder. In some women the pain is excruciating. Many develop a "frozen shoulder" because movement makes the pain worse; they protect the affected arm to the point that they lose mobility in the joint. This phenomenon is more common in women who remember severe postoperative pain and whose memory of how terrible it was increases with time. Understandably, these women eventually became sadder and more anxious than other patients who did not have this syndrome.

During the middle of the menstrual cycle, when progesterone levels are high, women's brains have reduced activation patterns in response to painful stimuli. Progesterone, which is also at high levels when a woman is nursing a baby, is a sedating and anesthetizing hormone. In fact, the chemical structure of some anesthetics (alphaxolone, for example) is very much like that of progesterone. This sedating aspect is one way the body prepares a woman for bearing a child and nursing a newborn. Testosterone, for its part, mutes men's experience of pain, which is one of the reasons that as men age and testosterone levels decrease, they become more sensitive to painful stimuli. (Testosterone's dampening effect on pain perception is probably a coping maneuver to minimize the pain of physical combat for men that has evolved over millennia.)

Sometimes, for reasons scientists aren't entirely sure of, hormones seem to exacerbate pain rather than mute it. A recent study showed that women who use birth control pills are more likely to have pain in the temporomandibular joint (TMJ, the joint connecting the jaw to the skull) than women who do not use them. In postmenopausal women, estrogen and, to a lesser extent, progesterone use significantly increases the risk for TMJ syndrome. The important point here is that exogenous hormones modulate the experience of pain, and women should know this when they agree to use birth control pills or HRT.

THE BRAIN AND PAIN

The brain's organized system to receive, modulate, and react to painful stimuli is complex: essentially, it consists of four interactive components. The first receives the stimulus and transmits it to the brain, where the second integrates the activity of the parts of the brain that identify the nature of the stimulus, assess its importance, and generate an appropriate emotional response to it. The third component then telegraphs a message to the systems in the body that are under automatic or involuntary control, like breathing and digestion (which is why pain changes heart rate and blood pressure). Finally, the fourth component provides feedback about changes in those systems to the brain, so that those changes can be modified or stabilized.

The central networks of these components may be importantly modified by hormones: in adult female rats, the portion of the brain called the locus coeruleus, which is concerned with arousal and pain modulation, is bigger and has more cells than in male rats. If a female rat receives testosterone on the first day of her life, this difference never develops.

Male rats are more sensitive to morphine than female rats, who seem to have their own "built-in" nonopioid pain-killer, which is related at least in part to estrogen production. Female rats secrete more of these chemicals during the birth of pups than at other times, which may make delivery less painful for them.

There may be important gender differences in the sites of the brain that are involved with the perception of and physiological response to pain. For example, MRI imaging has shown that in both men and women, if the bowels are distended to the point of being painful, the same areas of the brain are activated. But when men and women with irritable bowel syndrome are given the same stimulus, *different* areas of the brain are activated between the two sexes. Why is the pain from IBS encoded differently for women than for men? What does this mean for pain control or for the treatment of IBS? Scientists still don't know the answers.

OTHER GENDER DIFFERENCES IN
THE BODY'S RESPONSE TO PAIN

Men's and women's responses to pain also differ physiologically. For example, men in pain are more likely to experience a rise in blood pressure, whereas women in pain experience an accelerated heart rate more than do men. In cases of severe pain (produced in one study by occluding blood supply to the arm), women's blood pressure rises only a little or not at all, and as pain is increased, their blood pressure falls. But in men blood pressure rises as soon as pain is experienced, and it continues to do so as the pain increases. These findings suggest not simply a physiological but an emotional and/or behavioral component to pain response. This is very useful information for the gender-specific treatment of pain. In the recovery room after surgery, anesthesiologists traditionally gauge the amount of pain that needs treatment *by monitoring the patient for an increase in blood pressure* rather than heart rate. While this is a good index of discomfort in men, it is not as useful for monitoring postoperative pain in women.

Males who are stressed by intellectual challenges, like a school examination, secrete more adrenaline and cortisol (the stress hormones) than do females. In men, moreover, these hormones also seem to evoke feelings of accomplishment and triumph. Women in the same situation, however, produce less stress hormones and report more feelings of failure and anxiety. The stress response begins in the brain and works through the pituitary gland to stimulate the adrenal glands to produce these stress hormones, a process called *activation of the hypothalamic-pituitary axis.* R. B. Fillingim and William Maixner at the University of North Carolina in Chapel Hill have a very interesting idea of why noxious stimuli activate this axis in men more than in women; they hypothesize that the difference is an important result of evolutionary selection, because activating the axis brings practically all levels of the reproductive process to a halt.[3] They point out that stress-induced analgesia (pain relief) is much less effective in females after ovulation, suggesting that this cyclic suppression of the activation of the axis preserves fertility.

GENDER AND PAINFUL DISEASES

Headache

In a comprehensive recent review of gender differences in chronic headache, Dawn A. Marcus at the University of Pittsburgh observes that the incidence of simple chronic headache was equal in both sexes, but women had worse headache-related *emotional distress,* and men had more headache-related *disability* (they were less able to work and function at daily tasks than women).[4] A combination of depression and anxiety was identified in 75 percent of female sufferers but in only 25 percent of the men; 45 percent of all patients, regardless of gender, had anxiety. Dietary restrictions and regularization of eating patterns were more helpful to women than to men. Findings like these, that women's pain may stem more often from depression and can be managed more easily with simple diet adjustments, will prove valuable in our attempts to develop gender-specific strategies for pain management.

Some kinds of pain seem quite specifically associated with the female sex. A certain type of susceptibility to migraine headaches that runs in families, for example, stems from a defect on the X chromosome, which may help to explain why migraines are more frequent in women than in men. Migraine headaches are definitely more frequent in women (15 to 17 percent of all females have them) than in men (3 to 6 percent). Interestingly, this difference does not develop until puberty; until then, boys and girls seem to be equally affected, although the incidence in boys is maximal at five years of age and in girls at twelve. The difference begins to decrease again when adults reach middle age and tends to disappear as people age further. Migraines are associated with depression, and some scientists believe that the increased incidence in women is related to the fact that depression in women is more common.

Hormones too are probably to blame. Migraines worsen in many women with the menstrual period, probably because estrogen levels decrease at that time. In fact, 14 percent of women sufferers have migraines only in connection with their menstrual periods. Interestingly, it seems to be the change in estrogen concentrations, more than the low levels, that triggers migraine. Before low levels of estrogen will cause a headache, women have to be exposed to it in high levels (estrogen priming). If estrogen levels are chronically low (as they are in the postmenopausal period), headaches disappear. High estrogen levels are associated with high levels of one of the chemicals in the brain, 5-hydroxy tryptamine (5-HT), which inhibits the pain of headaches; when estrogen levels fall, so does 5-HT and the result is a migraine. Because of the potentiating effect of estrogen on migraine, 40 percent of women who suffer from migraines and use birth control medication will have an increase in symptoms. This may persist for as long as a year after stopping oral contraceptives. Progesterone-only contraception, on the other hand, increases symptoms only about 3 percent in migraine sufferers, although it is associated with other (tension-type) headaches in 25 percent of women who use this method. Pregnancy, because it provides the mother with stable estrogen levels, usually helps headache; it is the cyclicity of estrogen levels that cause the problem. In postmenopausal women, the introduction of HRT may cause an increase in the severity and frequency of headaches; this is usually handled by using a constant estrogen dosage instead of cyclic therapy.

Menstrual migraines can be treated quite effectively with low-dose estrogen patches four days before and for the first three days of the menstrual period.

In contrast to migraine headaches, cluster headaches are more frequent (by 4 to 7.5 times) in men. These intensely painful headaches occur in groups or clusters; between a series of attacks, patients are peculiarly symptom free. These headaches too are thought to be a result of hormonal dysregulation—in this case, a relatively low concentration of testosterone, caused by an impaired ability to make testosterone in response to luteinizing hormone (LH). An excess of epidermal growth hormone is known to impair the response of the gonads to LH and is thought to be the reason for cluster headaches as well as the peculiar lionlike facial appearance, known as leonine facies, of men who have them.

Osteoarthritis

This wear-and-tear disease of the joints affects 40 percent of middle-age adults and 70 percent of those over sixty. The specific joints are not affected equally in men and women: females are twice as likely to have arthritic knees than are men, but arthritis of the hips is equal in the sexes.

Francis J. Keefe, a psychologist at Ohio University, studied sex differences in the pain men and women feel with osteoarthritis. He found that women show a unique approach to the discomfort: 40 percent more females than males complained about their pain, and they were also more proactive than men in talking to others about it, asking for help from friends and families, and seeking distractions and counseling. This resulted in less depression in women than in men after a day of particularly disturbing pain. When subjects were shown videotapes of their spouses performing ordinary tasks, women were also better than men at identifying pain in their spouses. (The increased sensitivity of wives was only to their own husbands, by the way; it didn't extend to anyone else!) When Keefe studied the interactions of spouses with osteoarthritis when they were together, he found that the women tended to complain and give nonverbal clues about their discomfort (wincing, grimacing, and so on), whereas husbands encouraged their arthritic wives with humor as a supportive strategy.

Coronary Artery Disease

Coronary artery disease is a very interesting illness for gender-specific medicine because so many features of it differ between the sexes (see Chapter 5); one of the most important is pain. The famous Framingham Heart Study, which began in 1948 and traced the natural history of CAD in the population of a small New England town, was the first study to point out differences between men's and women's experience of the disease. Doctors have long known that chest pain in women is much less well correlated with demonstrable disease of the coronary arteries when patients come to cardiac catheterization: 50 percent of women with chest pain show no disease in the large arteries supplying the heart, while the figure for men is only 17 percent. On the other hand, this does not mean the disease is less serious for women than men: more women than men *have no pain at all with their heart attacks,* these are called *silent myocardial infarctions* (SMIs). One in five women has a very unusual but consistent presentation: a constellation of pain in the upper abdomen or back, extreme shortness of breath, and profuse sweating.

The disconnect between severe chest pain and actual CAD is most marked in younger women; severe chest pain appeared in pre-menopausal women with high estrogen levels and in postmenopausal women on HRT. At this writing, The National Institutes of Health is completing a four-year study of the nature and cause of chest pain in women (the Women's Ischemia Syndrome Evaluation, or WISE, study); results should be forthcoming soon and will help doctors iden tify and treat the cause of chest pain in women much more accurately. Most physicians who treat women for chest pain believe that in a substantial number of patients the pain is caused by *spasm of the heart's small muscular arteries.* Such spasm can't be visualized by cardiac catheterization, in which only the largest vessels at the surface of the heart are filled with dye and examined for dangerous deposits of plaque.

Recently David Sheps and his colleagues at East Tennessee University reported on their detailed investigation of what *produces* angina (chest pain brought on by emotion or exertion) in men and women.[5] The subjects agreed to endure physical and emotional challenges on two different days and report their responses. Women's complaints of chest pain were *more frequent on a day when they experienced mental stress* (public speaking) *and on an ordinary day* than on a day of physical stress (riding a stationary bicycle). Like the rats I've described earlier in this chapter, women turned out to have lower levels than men of beta-endorphins—the chemicals in the brain that soothe and comfort and that increase in response to pain.

Reproductive Organs

Both men and women experience chronic pain in the reproductive organs, but the medications that help men don't work as well in women. Ursula Wesselmann at Johns Hopkins University School of Medicine compared 25 women with chronic noncancerous pelvic pain with 25 men with chronic nonmalignant testicular pain and gave each patient one of four different types of medication: an antidepressant, an anticonvulsant, an opioid, or a membrane-stabilizing agent.[6] All of these medications worked better to relieve women's pain—except for antidepressants, which worked better in men: 9 out of 11 men improved with antidepressant medication, compared with only 4 out of 25 women.

Other interesting data emerged from Wesselmann's study:

- Women and men both found the pain hard to localize but severe enough at times to make them nauseated and sweaty.
- Both sexes found it hard to discuss pain in these areas with a doctor and as a result delayed seeking help for their discomfort.
- In women, the intensity of chronic pelvic pain may have no relationship to the physical source of the problem; the small site of endometriosis in the uterus, for example, can cause significant discomfort.
- Women have a 5 percent lifetime risk of chronic pelvic pain and a 20 percent lifetime risk of pelvic inflammatory disease; in both cases the pain can persist even when the acute infection has been cured.
- Men suffer chronic pain (that lasts more than three months) in their testes in their late thirties; in a third of these men, no disorder is apparent, but in the other two-thirds, bicycle accidents, vasectomies, infections, and tumors are triggering causes.

Fibromyalgia

One of the most poorly understood disorders that doctors face in practice is fibromyalgia (FM), which is what I call a "wastebasket illness."* Like chronic fatigue syndrome, it is not a flight of a patient's imagination: it causes life-disrupting discomfort and is extraordinarily difficult to treat. Researchers know almost nothing about its cause or where the symptoms come from. Some important recent advances in our under-

---

* "Wastebasket illness" is a commonly used phrase for diseases doctors don't understand and many do not believe are genuine illnesses.

standing of fibromyalgia, which occurs in nine times as many women as men, come from Laurence A. Bradley at the University of Alabama.[7] He studied 66 women being treated in a fibromyalgia clinic. All had had more than three months of widespread body pain and had increased pain in response to pressure in at least eleven of the eighteen points that are considered characteristically sensitive in FM. Bradley documented several interesting facts:

- FM patients found a pressure stimulus of any given strength more painful than did healthy women.
- *FM patients' cerebrospinal fluid contained more P substance (a chemical involved in transmitting the message of pain to the brain) than did that of healthy women.*
- The areas of the brain critical to the experience of pain were different in FM patients than in healthy women.
- More FM patients had been diagnosed with psychiatric illnesses (anxiety disorder, depression, and the like) than healthy women.

Temporomandibular Disorder

Temporomandibular disorder (TMD) involves pain in the temporomandibular joint, which joins the lower jaw (the mandible) to the skull, and in the surrounding muscles. It affects seven times as many women as men. It is quite common, affecting as many as one in four young adult females, according to William Maixner at the University of North Carolina at Chapel Hill. Several aspects of the disease are reminiscent of the kinds of symptoms endured by FM patients:

- TMD patients feel painful stimuli anywhere in the body much more intensely than do healthy people.[8]
- When healthy people have a toothache, a tight tourniquet on the arm lessens or eliminates the tooth pain. (The painful impulses from the arm "jam the highway" to the brain so that impulses from the tooth are blocked.) But when Maixner tried this maneuver in patients with TMD, two-thirds of them had either no change or an increase in their tooth pain!

- FM and TMD may overlap, because 75 percent of FM patients have TMD, and the latter may actually be an early stage of fibromyalgia.

MEN AND WOMEN IN PAIN: SHOULD DOCTORS TREAT THEM BOTH THE SAME WAY?

As we saw in Chapter 3, each medication has its own particular pharmacokinetics, which may vary according to an individual patient's gender, genotype, and other factors. Premenopausal women, for example, do not absorb medications in a consistent way. During midcycle their gastric absorption of alcohol and aspirin is less efficient, and the intestinal transit time of any ingested substance slows down. This is also true during pregnancy and when women take hormonal supplements or birth control pills. Levels of proteins that bind a drug like lidocaine (an anesthetic given by injection) are generally lower in women than in men, and less of the drug is bound in a female patient taking birth control pills (which compete for binding with the lidocaine). The more a drug binds to carrier-proteins, the less effective it generally is.

Men and women metabolize drugs in significantly different ways (see Chapter 3) because of the sex-specific characteristics of the liver's cytochrome P450 system, which purifies the blood. Birth control pills can intensify the effect of some pain medications by lengthening the time they remain in the body. Other medicines, like the sedative and anticonvulsant drug mephobarbital, are processed more quickly by younger men than by women and older men, as a function of younger men's higher testosterone levels.

Males, as I've said, seem to be more sensitive than women to morphine. And for some reason, nonsteroidal anti-inflammatories (NSAIDs) like ibuprofen (Advil) are less likely to reduce pain in women than in men, although they reduce inflammation equally in both sexes. So the pain relief a woman experiences from an NSAID may be a consequence of its effect on inflammation more than the drug's direct action on her pain.

Such data make it important for a physician to consider a woman's age, weight, and body composition, as well as whether she is taking birth control pills, before prescribing pain medication or anesthesia for her. If her pain is recurrent and cyclic, a preemptive strike might be useful, starting pain medication in advance of the predicted discomfort or the time when the pain is expected to be worse. A fixed regimen might not be the most useful strategy, since many painful conditions worsen during the menstrual period. So pain medication might be increased automatically just before menses begin.

Medicines used during and after surgical procedures should be carefully chosen on the basis of the patient's sex. Women experience more muscle discomfort and headache after surgery, which may well be related to a muscle relaxant used during surgery called succinyl choline; this drug is associated with more muscle pain in women than in men in the first days after recovery from surgery.

Finally, education and attitude may be among the most useful tools we have for pain management. Lamaze classes for women and their husbands on how to get through labor, for example, have proven very helpful. In general, women are more willing than men to verbalize their concerns and respond to communication and teaching from their health care providers. Doctors should make an extra effort to teach male patients about their treatment options, especially when it seems that situational changes (like finding suitable help) or adjunctive therapies (like meditation or massage) might help recovery or at least lessen the intensity of discomfort.

Throughout the pain-management process, physicians have to consider their own attitudes toward pain. Many doctors are more likely to discount women's complaints than men's, out of a conviction that women are simply less able to bear discomfort than men. These prejudices are hard to expunge. In fact, in my experience, most physicians avoid scrutinizing their own abilities to be objective and helpful to patients. One of the first—and last—chances that the health care system has to help doctors improve their interpersonal skills and correct harmful and destructive attitudes to patients is during their medical school training and immediately after graduation from medical school, when they are house officers on a hospital staff. In addition to the spoken instructions of older physicians, the example provided by supervising doctors as they deal with patients become very important in molding the sensitivity and empathy of young trainees.

WHAT DOES THE NEW SCIENCE MEAN FOR YOU?

I am planning elective (nonemergency) surgery. Does it matter what phase of my menstrual cycle I'm in when I have the operation?

You might have not only less pain but a better response to medication in midcycle than just before or during your menstrual period. Ask your doctor to consider your monthly cycle in scheduling the procedure.

Every time I menstruate, I get a terrible headache. Why? Can I do anything about it?

Menstrual migraines are not a mystery: they occur because of the sudden drop in estrogen that precedes the beginning of menstruation. Often the temporary use of an estrogen patch just before and during the first few days of a menstrual cycle will help.

Which is likely to be more effective in relieving pain from my infected finger, Tylenol or Advil?

If you are a woman and your pain is caused by an infection, you are more likely to get relief from a nonsteroidal agent like aspirin or ibuprofen than from acetaminophen. Inflammation is a bigger component of a response to infection in women than in men, so a drug that specifically lessens inflammation is likely to be more helpful for pain relief.

My doctor told me I couldn't be having a heart attack, because I was having back pain and not chest pain. Yet I was terribly short of breath, nause-

ated, and sweating profusely. In fact, testing in the ER proved I had a heart attack. Why was my pain in such an unusual place?

The place you experienced pain was not unusual for a woman: one out of five women with acute heart attack (myocardial infarction) has pain in the epigastrium (upper abdomen) and not under the breastbone, which is the classic site for discomfort in men. Sex-specific differences in the anatomy of the nervous system produce gender-specific variations in the sites of pain; often it can be relatively remote from the organ that's injured. If you suspect you're having a heart attack, insist that it be ruled out by proper testing before you agree to leave the emergency room!

I couldn't convince my doctor to give me enough medicine for pain just after I had major abdominal surgery; he said he saw no indication to increase my dose over what he'd already given me. What criterion was he using to decide?

Probably it was the fact that your blood pressure didn't rise when you began to feel more pain. In men, the level of pain is mirrored by a rise in blood pressure. For women patients, informed anesthesiologists follow the heart rate rather than the blood pressure to monitor the severity of pain.

Pain medication seems to wear off in my husband sooner than it does for me. Is he just a wimp?

Decidedly not: men and women process many pain-killers, anesthetics, and other medicines differently. Some drugs bind to fat cells, and women have more body fat than men. You might absorb more of the drug than your husband does because everything, including food, moves through women's digestive tracts more slowly than through men's. Some of the difference may be genetic: a small percentage of men can't metabolize codeine properly, and so they get little or no pain relief from the medication.

The time in your menstrual cycle and whether you take oral con-traceptives could also influence the efficacy of a pain-relieving drug: some hormones compete in the liver for the sites used to process med-icines and make them available to the body. If one pain-reliever works less well depending on your cycle, for example, let your doctor know so that she can choose another type of analgesic for you.

I've noticed a really painful ache in my jaw recently. What should I tell my doctor that might be relevant to why this is happening?

One thing you might want to mention is whether you are taking prescribed oral contraceptives: women who use them are more likely to have temporomandibular joint pain than those who don't.

After an exhausting fight with my husband, I notice that he's much less depressed than I am—I feel exhausted and anxious. Is this sociology (he simply doesn't care as much if we're getting along) or biology?

It could be both. Both sexes, when stressed, secrete the stress hor-mones adrenaline and cortisol, but men secrete more than women. In men, these hormones are more likely to evoke feelings of triumph and success; for women, the effect is to lower self-esteem and increase anxiety.

When my husband had a tooth pulled yesterday, I offered him one of the pain-killers my dentist gave me when I had my own extraction. It worked fine in my case, but my husband didn't get much relief. Is it because he's big-ger than I am and needs a bigger dose?

It depends on the medication. The brain has two kinds of receptors for analgesic drugs: the μ-opioid and the k-opioid. Women get a much better effect from drugs that interact with the latter. Several medicines dispensed by dentists work better in women; three of them are penta-zocine (Talwin), nalbuphine (Nubain), and butorphanol (Stadol).

CHAPTER 10

Sexual Dysfunction

⁓

ROBABLY NO HUMAN function is more complex than sex. Intercourse can be a profoundly engaging experience that involves all of our
faculties, or it can be a trivial encounter that's over in less than a minute
and of no significance at all—or worse, even distasteful. The very phrases
we use to name sex connote a wide range of involvement. *Making love* is
quite different conceptually from *having sex;* one implies genuine emotional engagement, and the other describes purely physical gratification.

Quite apart from the difficulties in measuring aspects of sexual
experience, the physiology of sex is now understood quite well. Because
of our better appreciation of how the body changes during the various
phases of desire, arousal, climax, and resolution, we also understand
what can go wrong and cause sexual dysfunction (SD). It is different in
many ways for men and women, and even the aging process affects sex
for the two genders in unique ways.

WHAT IS SEXUAL DYSFUNCTION?

Psychiatrists divide sexual problems into four categories:

- *Problems with desire or libido.* These problems can be very different for men and women. Men's libido is more easily triggered than

women's by external cues like visual stimulation, for example. For women, *sexual aversion disorder* (SAD) is a more common problem, in which the idea of sex provokes feelings of disgust or anxiety. Often, and perhaps not surprisingly, this disorder is associated with previous sexual abuse or trauma.

• *Problems with arousal.* In men this problem is expressed as failure to achieve or maintain an erection. The prevalence increases with age; 15 percent of men between forty and seventy have minimal impairment, 25 percent have moderate impairment, and 10 percent have complete impotence.[1] Youth doesn't guarantee erectile competence: between ages nineteen and forty-nine, 5 to 10 percent of men have problems, and the figure jumps to 20 percent for men fifty to fifty-nine.[2] Almost every investigator to whom I have talked about this subject agrees that women can exhibit all the physical signs of sexual arousal but *not experience the fact that they are aroused!* This is only one reason that arousal disorders are much harder to diagnose in women than in men. The diagnosis depends on the patient's experience of arousal; the presence of physical signs of sexual arousal is not relevant. Whereas erection is a reliable indicator of arousal in men, we still have no reliable indicator of arousal in women.

• *Problems with orgasm.* Most experts in the field of sexuality believe that women are more likely to have satisfactory sex lives than men. In fact, some scientists attribute orgasmic disorder in women either to negative sexual counseling or training as they were growing up or to restrictive social and cultural views of women and sexuality. Some women are *truly* unable to climax, no matter what the situation. (Many women who don't climax during intercourse can do so if they masturbate or if their partner brings them to orgasm by oral or manual stimulation.) A physician usually needs great delicacy and more than a few visits from the patient to decide why this is the case and, if it really is, what combination of treatments to knit together to help the patient. Unfortunately, doctors and patients don't talk about sex as easily as about other issues. A telephone survey of American adults found that younger women don't talk to their doctors about sexual problems because they fear that the *doctors* will be embarrassed by the issue—and won't know how to solve them!

• *Pain with sex, for females.* This is a problem for 10 to 15 percent of North American women; younger women have more difficulty than older women.*

HOW COMMON IS SD?

One of my favorite quotes on the subject of sex comes from Sandra Leiblum, the director of the Center for Sexual and Marital Health in Piscataway, New Jersey: "Although people are bombarded daily with sexual references, pictures, articles, and exploits of both famous and infamous individuals, actual sexual comfort and effortless sexual performance tend to be rather rare. In fact, sexual problems and complaints in both sexes are ubiquitous."[3]

Scientists who are studying sexual function agree with Leiblum. In a study of "normal" couples, Ellen Frank, of the University of Pittsburgh, found that although the subjects considered themselves happily married, a significant proportion of both men (14 percent) and women (15 percent) felt that their sex lives were seriously lacking. Forty percent of men had problems with erection and ejaculation (usually early); and in almost 70 percent of cases, women had difficulty with arousal or climaxing.[4] Other investigators have found equally high numbers of people dissatisfied with their sex lives: in one study, 15 percent of men and 35 percent of women had inhibited sexual desire, 10 to 20 percent of men had erectile problems, and 35 percent suffered from premature ejaculation. Five to 30 percent of women had problems with orgasm.[5] In general, studies indicate that about 43 percent of women and 31 percent of men have issues with sexual function.

As doctors' ability—and willingness—to understand sexual function improves, largely due to the pioneering work of scientists like Masters, Johnson, and Kaplan, we have learned not only the details of how men's and women's bodies respond to sexual stimulation but the reasons why sexual function can be less than ideal. For example, we

---

* Pain associated with sex is not limited to pain on actual intercourse. *Noncoital sexual pain* occurs simply on being sexually stimulated.

know now that aging doesn't mean the automatic loss of interest in sex—far from it, in fact. The simple fact of menopause doesn't mean that a woman abandons all thought of sex: satisfactory experiences with her partner can continue well into oldest age. Properly understood and treated, many of the obstacles associated with aging (and its concomitant decrease in hormones) can be treated and eliminated.

MENOPAUSE AND ANDROPAUSE: "CHANGE OF LIFE" IS NOT FOR WOMEN ONLY!

The Massachusetts Women's Health Study II provided important information about changes in women's sexual function over time as a function of menopause. The 200 women in the study, who ranged in age from fifty-one to sixty-one, reported three things: a lessened desire for sex, a conviction that sexual activity falls off as people age, and diminished arousal compared with the time when they were forty and premenopausal.

Both men and women have less sexual activity as they age, but the reasons are different: men have more difficulty attaining and sustaining an erection (erectile dysfunction), while women more often lack a suitable partner.

From age thirty-five onward, sexual interest is thought to be higher in men than in women, but this may be incorrect. For example, a woman over thirty-five may be paired with an older partner who has difficulty with erection and therefore may lose some enthusiasm for initiating sexual contact. Men may be more reluctant than women to admit a decline of interest in sex. One thing seems to be true, though: men's desire consistently declines as they age, but women's does not! If the opportunity is there, a woman can respond to and enjoy sexual contact well into old age.

Some of the reported decline in sexual activity in postmenopausal women may be cultural: an apparent bias against sex without emotional involvement for females and a notion that younger males are not appropriate partners for older females. Both ideas limit opportunity for women: I have explored these attitudes with my patients and find that in fact many women enjoy sex without profound emotional involvement, particularly when they are older and surer of themselves. The notion of younger men as partners seems less easy to accept, but they might make as least as satisfying sexual companions as same-aged men. In fact, many younger men are interested in confident, attractive older women. The conventional he-is-older-than-she "ideal" should be routinely challenged in discussions of sexuality with both sexes.

Men are also affected by *andropause,* a phenomenon similar to menopause that is also due to an aging-related decline in hormonal levels, in this case testosterone. Some doctors believe that andropause is not as dramatic as menopause and occurs over a longer period of time; but others think that the aging process is quite similar in character—and in pace—for both sexes. Like women, men also experience impaired memory and inability to think clearly, and they suffer changes in mood as testosterone levels drift downward. They have hot flashes, decreased sexual desire, and less vigorous sexual performance as they age. Many men benefit from testosterone-replacement therapy.

HOW HORMONES DEFINE SEXUAL EXPERIENCE IN MEN AND WOMEN

Hormones in Women

The ovaries and to a lesser extent the adrenal glands are the factories that produce the three principal hormones that make women women: estrogen, progesterone, and testosterone. During the time when we are able to have children (from puberty, when the ovaries begin to be active, to menopause, when they no longer produce the eggs from which children can develop), the brain regulates the production of all three hormones in a cyclic, rhythmic pattern of ovarian stimulation. In the loop between the brain and the ovaries, the chief control center is the pituitary gland, which sits like a pea on a stalk at the base of the brain. The philosopher Descartes thought the pituitary was the seat of the soul; when I was a medical student first reading about the protean functions that this tiny, highly specialized organ accomplishes, I wondered if Descartes had been right!

Among other things, the pituitary gland sends two hormones into the bloodstream to direct the activity of the gonads: one is luteinizing hormone (LH) and the other is follicle-stimulating hormone (FSH). Ovaries have two different kinds of cells: one type responds to LH and makes a variety of androgens (male hormones; *androgen* literally means "male-creating"), including testosterone. The other type responds to FSH; these cells have the enzyme aromatase (see Chapter 2), which converts testosterone to estrogen. Women have a relatively higher concentration of estrogen than men, but in both the source for the "female" hormone is testosterone. The other important thing to know about hormones is that both sexes have all three; it is only the concentrations of the hormones that are different between males and females.

Both estrogen and testosterone affect sexual function in women. The female libido (or sexual desire) is largely under the control of testosterone, while the changes in the body that accompany arousal and climax are due to the action of estrogen. Before menopause, the ovaries produce most of the androgens that support women's sexual interest or desire, but after menopause, even though their bodies continue to produce some androgens (like the much-discussed dihydroepiandrosterone [DHEA]), levels of testosterone drift slowly downward, and as they grow older, many women experience a banking of the fires of sexual desire. Some women lose most or all of their interest in sex as they age; others, for a variety of reasons, continue to seek out and enjoy sexual activity, even in very old age. As physicians' sophistication increases, they are learning to test postmenopausal women for testosterone deficiency; supplementing this hormone not only increases libido but improves muscle bulk, restores flagging energy, and can stimulate the growth of testosterone-dependent hair follicles like those in the pubic and axillary areas. It also can improve dry skin and brittle nails.

The other important change that comes with aging in women is that the ovaries stop making estrogen; what estrogen continues to circulate comes from the fat cells, which convert adrenal gland androgens to estrogen. (When postmenopausal women lose a great deal of weight, they also lose stored hormones, and so they begin to have signs of more intense estrogen deficiency. Several of my patients who went on punishing diets began to have hot flashes and sleep disturbances again, just as they had immediately before and during their menopause!) How much weight is "right" for older women? There may be a very good evolutionary reason why postmenopausal women slowly gain weight: the added fat may be an important source of extra estrogen (or estradiol, the active form of estrogen). In contrast to estrogen, ovarian production of androgens continues after menopause, but less actively.

The changes in estrogen concentration that come with aging have important consequences on women's bodies:

• The lining of the vagina gets thinner and drier. The glands that produce the secretions that lubricate the vagina and its entrance become smaller and less active. This not only makes the vagina an easier target for infection but can make intercourse painful.

• The lining of the urethra (the short passage from the bladder to the outside world) thins too; not only does this make urinary tract infections more common, but it can result in a loss of urine when we cough or sneeze (stress incontinence) or a sudden, unwanted, and uncontrollable overflow of urine when the bladder is full. Patients with atrophy of the urethral lining complain of always feeling the urge to urinate, even when they don't have a full bladder, and they visit the bathroom far more often than when they were younger—with much less efficiency per visit!

• The pubic hair thins, the tissue underneath it (the mons pubis) flattens out, the folds of tissue that protect the vaginal and urethral openings (the labia majora) lose thickness, and the vagina becomes less elastic.

• During the excitement or arousal phase of sex, the skin flushes less than it did before, the opening of the urethra dilates, the breasts do not swell with stimulation, lubrication is delayed or absent, and the vagina does not expand sufficiently to accommodate the penis.

• Finally, the lower level of hormones in the older woman may produce difficulty in achieving orgasm and a disturbing loss of intensity of orgasm when it does occur. Some women say that the contractions of their uterus, which are part of climax, become painful rather than pleasurable. Most aging women report fewer and less intense orgasm than they experienced when they were younger. Happily, estrogen and, in some circumstances, testosterone replacement therapy carefully tailored to the needs of the individual woman can improve or abolish many of these changes.

The two most common problems women experience with sexual function are loss of desire and painful intercourse. Loss of desire is probably more complicated to treat, but HRT is an important antidote for both problems. Doctors can measure estrogen levels in the blood to decide whether HRT is warranted. An estradiol level below 25 to 50 picograms per milliliter can be the cause of vaginal dryness and pain on intercourse. Serum levels of estrogen can be deceiving, though, because many unrelated factors can cause a false reading (like how much binding protein for a hormone is circulating in the blood). A more reliable way for a doctor to determine whether a woman has adequate estrogen is to examine a sample of her vaginal lining under the microscope: a well-estrogenized lining is many layers thick.

Paradoxically, estrogen-replacement therapy *may actually lessen sexual desire because it increases the levels of sex-hormone-binding globulin in the blood,* which sops up testosterone and makes it unavailable for use! Women who experience this effect should have testosterone supplementation as well as estrogen replacement therapy.

In women the association between a loss of libido or sexual desire and abnormally low levels of testosterone is incontrovertible. But before you decide that your hormones are out of whack or deficient, remember that *the circumstances of our lives also reduce (or enhance) sexual feelings and desire.* Many of my women patients complain that they no longer are interested in sexual exchange with their husbands. I always ask them if they have enjoyed a recent vacation alone with him, far from the concerns of everyday life, including children, work, and financial concerns. If they have, and they say their sexuality was "like a second honeymoon," their problem is clearly situational, not hormonal. If a woman loves her spouse, though, and privacy and lack of distraction aren't the issues, hormone supplementation might help—it's worth a careful look.

Measuring hormone levels is not an easy task, and testosterone is no exception. Neither is it easy to decide what levels are *too* low in a woman. Most experts agree that a patient *who has adequate levels of estrogen and progesterone* should be considered for testosterone replacement when she has low libido, decreased motivation, fatigue, and a reduced or absent sense of well-being. (Note that all of these symptoms are also typical of depression, however!) The best way to assess the adequacy of testosterone levels is to measure the ratio of testosterone to sex-hormone-binding globulin (SHBG), or measure the level of free testosterone; if it is in the lowest third of the normal reproductive female range, a woman can be considered testosterone deficient. Usually, testosterone deficiency is most common in women when the ovaries fail completely or are surgically removed, since in women the principal source of androgen (of which testosterone is an example) is the ovaries. (There is a surge of testosterone production in the ovaries in midcycle.)

Taking HRT or using an oral contraceptive can lower testosterone levels because they increase levels of SHBG (which binds free hormones and makes them unavailable for use) and suppress the luteinizing hormone, produced by the pituitary, that stimulates the ovaries to produce testosterone. Taking steroids also lowers testosterone production because steroids suppress adrenal gland function, which is also a source of testosterone.

By what mechanisms can testosterone improve the sex lives of women? It works in a combination of ways. Androgens can act directly on androgen receptors, or they can be converted to estrogen by aromatase in the tissues or by lowering SHBG and increasing the free circulating concentrations of all the hormones. Experts believe all are important in heightening sexuality.

When estrogen and testosterone replacement are combined, studies show that women taking both hormones had less nausea, less breast tenderness, and less pelvic congestion than those taking estrogen alone. Most doctors now believe that testosterone is the most important agent for improving libido, while both estrogen and testosterone are involved in satisfactory arousal and orgasm.

Hormones in Men

I've already discussed the fact that in men testosterone levels decrease with age, and that this decrease not only has an enormous impact on men's sexual function but produces a series of physical changes very similar to those that women experience after menopause. Although men have more difficulty getting and sustaining an erection as they age, less than 5 percent of erectile dysfunction (ED) is thought to be caused by testosterone deficiency. The problem may in fact be due to illness or medications. Physicians should take care to note the side effects and interactions of the medications they prescribe and adjust the dosages if ED becomes a problem.

Other aging-related changes in hormone levels affect function too, particularly in men. Growth hormone decreases more in men than in women. When we are younger, growth hormone protects us against loss of neurons or nerve cells, stems the tide of cell death in our tissues, and prevents osteoporosis. But as we age, lower levels increase the amount of SHBG in the blood that binds (and makes unavailable) our sex hormones.

Melatonin is another important hormone that decreases in both sexes with aging: melatonin regulates the periodic functions of our lives like sleep and wake cycles. These are called our circadian rhythms, and decreased levels of this hormone is one reason sleep is for fewer hours and more difficult to sustain for reasonable periods of time as we grow older. In rats, at least, resupplying them with melatonin restores natural sleep.

PHYSICAL CAUSES OF SEXUAL DYSFUNCTION

Bike Riding

Bike riding, whether for leisure or for serious sport, can produce serious sexual dysfunction in both men and women, for two reasons. One is the compression of the pelvic tissues against the bike's hard, narrow, and poorly padded seat. This can damage both the nerves that supply the genital area as well as the blood supply on which erection and orgasm depend. The second reason is injury from the impact of falling on the crossbar of a man's bike. The force of the impact can be as much as a quarter of a ton! The results of compression or injury can be very extensive; almost 13 percent of all bikers are impotent. More complain of some degree of ED, difficulty with orgasm, and more infections of the urinary tract than normal. Women bikers suffer the same results: a substantial number complain of perineal numbness, difficulty achieving orgasm, decreased orgasmic intensity, and urinary tract infection. Even stationary bikes (widely used for cardiovascular conditioning and weight loss regimens) are problematic and can cause real damage to sexual function and the urinary tract. Since it's estimated that there are 100 million bikers in the United States, everyone ought to consider this information when they decide on a recreational sport! Certainly serious bikers, who train and compete extensively, and mountain bikers, probably because of the bumpy terrain, suffer the most disability.

Sex, Illness, and Medicines

For men and women, illness can put a damper on sexual activity and even on the desire for sex. For example, someone who has had a heart attack may fear the exertion involved in resuming intimacy. For some reason, women are more susceptible to these kinds of feelings and fears and are less likely than men to resume normal sexual activity after recovery.

Diabetes can affect sexual function significantly. Interestingly, *treated* diabetics have more problems with ED and anorgasmia (lack of orgasm) than untreated diabetics. This may be related to the severity of disease as well as to side effects of the drugs used to treat diabetes. ED itself is due to two things: damage to the blood vessels supplying the pelvic and genital areas and injury to the nerves involved in sexual response. Failure to achieve erection is quite common in diabetic men.

Sexual dysfunction is also quite common in people with cardiovascular disease. Here again the cause might be the illness itself (arteriosclerosis can compromise blood supply to the areas involved in sexual function) or to the medications used to treat it. As is the case with diabetes, sexual dysfunction is more common in treated than in untreated cardiovascular patients. Of all the medicines used to treat cardiovascular disease, the worst offender is digitalis (almost always given as digoxin, whose commercial name is Lanoxin), because this medicine makes muscle cells contract with more force. While this effect is great for the heart muscle and helps cures congestive heart failure, it is terrible for the smooth muscle cells of the pelvic blood vessels and tissues, which have to relax during sexual arousal and climax. On the other hand, digoxin is a very useful drug for *priapism*, a disease in which men develop an erection that will not go away—a source of embarrassment and pain significant enough to drive many sufferers to visit emergency rooms.

Almost all of the medicines that doctors use to treat high blood pressure produce sexual dysfunction in both men and women. This problem often becomes really difficult, because finding the right combination of effective drugs to control hypertension may require months of experimentation (sometimes three or four medications are needed) only to produce ED in men and loss of libido in either sex. Sildenafil (Viagra) is useful in men who are impotent because of antihypertensive medicine, but women have no such solution, and doctors and patients alike are left with a real conundrum. Treating serious cardiovascular disease is more important to survival than correcting sexual dysfunction, but the quality of life can be significantly reduced when the price is sexual dysfunction.

Depression is another illness that kills sexual desire. About 60 percent of patients who have major depression experience a loss of interest in sex; in fact, it is the third most common symptom of depression, after sleep disturbances and early morning awakening. One study found an interesting difference between men and women: 68 percent of the men *but none of the women* with primary sexual dysfunction had an anxiety disorder.[6] This finding is unexpected, since anxiety disorders are more common in women, and the absence of an association between anxiety and sexual dysfunction in women is one of the surprising gender-specific findings that prompts new, as-yet-unanswered questions about the mechanics of biological function. Other important work has shown that depressed libido does not necessarily correlate with orgasmic dysfunction. R. J. Mathew and M. L. Weinman of Duke University found that although 31 percent of depressed men and women said they had blunted sexual desire, 22 percent had increased libido. Either the latter group were actually manic-depressives (during the manic phase of bipolar illness, many patients have an increase in sexuality), or they had a more intense need for closeness and emotional support than normal people.[7] Another interesting observation from a different study: 100 percent of women admitted to the hospital for alcoholism had problems with sexual function. Whether alcoholism was a primary cause or was the result of other factors like depression or chronic illness wasn't apparent from this study.

Unfortunately, some of the medicines used to treat depression just compound the problem of sexual dysfunction. The first widely used antidepressants, the tricyclics (like Elavil), and the monoamine oxidase inhibitors (like Desryl) as well as the SSRIs (Prozac and Paxil) can all intensify sexual dysfunction. About 43 percent of patients taking an SSRI are estimated to have problems of this nature, as a consequence not of the depression but of the medication. If a patient believes the medicine he or she is taking for sadness makes sexual dysfunction worse, the doctor has a few choices: give the patient a brief holiday from the drug, change it, or combine it with another medicine known to neutralize the sexual side effects.

Just as digoxin works as a cure for priapism, however, some of these drugs benefit the 30 percent of men who have premature ejaculation. SSRIs often cure the problem and are more and more widely used for this disorder. Unlike impotence (for which diabetes and cardiovascular disease are risk factors), premature ejaculation has no risk factors; it is *more common* within marriage (perhaps due to better feedback in a married state) and bears no relationship to age.

Peyronie's Disease

Peyronie's disease is a problem of poor healing of tears in the connective tissue that wraps around the penis; it can happen as a result of multiple small injuries during vigorous sexual activity, or from twisting an erect penis (causing a penile fracture). A plaque or scar forms at the point of injury, and the penis bends or is even deformed in three dimensions. (It can actually have a hourglass shape in some cases.) During arousal, the constriction or bend can prevent blood flow into the penis adequate for an erection. The only remedy is surgery, with straightening of the scarred penis; the procedure sometimes involves grafting the skin defect that results with strips of vein harvested from the patient's leg.

THE IMPACT OF SEXUAL ABUSE ON WOMEN'S SEXUAL ACTIVITY AND SELF-IMAGE

An important investigation into the impact of sexual abuse on women's sexuality was reported recently by Ann Kearney-Cooke and Diann M. Ackard of the Cincinnati Psychotherapy Institute.[8] Because childhood sexual abuse is widespread (it affects 20 to 30 percent of women and 10 to 15 percent of men), these investigators were interested in examining the late consequences of such abuse on women's images of themselves and on their sexual function. Eighty-four and a half percent of women felt that the abuse had had lasting negative effects, including more dissatisfaction with their bodies and overall with themselves as people. They were less successful at forming and maintaining intimate relationships with women who had not been abused and were less able to feel comfortable undressing in front of their sexual partners or making love with the lights on. Other, perhaps less anticipated late effects included a significantly increased incidence of eating disorders and *less use of contraceptives than other women*. In part, these effects may be due to a higher incidence of drug abuse and promiscuity in this population.

WHAT DOES THE NEW SCIENCE MEAN FOR YOU?

After years of a happy sexual relationship, my husband has suddenly stopped having erections. What's happened, and what can we do about it?

Erectile dysfunction is common, and its incidence increases with age; 20 percent of men between fifty and fifty-nine have problems. Besides aging, other causes of ED include:

- Depression. One of the first casualties of depression is sexual function. This problem can be compounded by the medications used to treat depression, particularly the SSRIs, which by the way are notorious for making orgasm very difficult to achieve in both males and females.
- Poor health. Illness can produce all kinds of sexual dysfunction, particularly ED. In particular, cardiovascular disease, diabetes, and alcohol abuse are likely to cause problems. (Incidentally, while a history of sexually transmitted disease seems to diminish women's libido, it doesn't affect that of men.)
- Medications. Besides the SSRIs, hypoglycemic agents (used to lower blood sugar in diabetics), antihypertensive medicines (used to lower blood pressure), and heart drugs may all produce ED.
- Stress. A drop in household income greater than 20 percent, for example, is associated with diminished libido, difficulty with arousal, and in particular, ED.
- Sexual abuse. This isn't exclusively a problem for women; men also endure sexual abuse as children. The abuse may have a particularly strong effect on sexual desire and performance if it occurred before puberty.

What should your husband do? First and most important, he should consult an internist or family physician for a complete assessment of his general health. If no cause for his problem is apparent, he should be referred to a specialist, probably a urologist, who is knowledgeable in diagnosing the reason for sexual dysfunction and treating it in both men and women. These physicians can monitor blood flow to the penis during sleep to see if erection ever occurs. If it does (or if your husband has a morning erection, even briefly), psychological factors are likely playing a role. They can also discuss some of the options open to him if he can't have an erection on his own: these include medications like sildenafil (Viagra) and alprostadil (Caverject), as well as penile pumps (which have to be surgically inserted).

What should you do? Make sure that some problem in your relationship of which you might not even be aware is causing the ED.

Often anger is acted out in the bedroom. Try to set aside some time for the two of you to talk—about your work, your lives, your relationship. Better communication will benefit all aspects of the relationship, including the romantic side. That done, be understanding and supportive, knowing what an important issue this is for most men's self-esteem.

I am a sixty-year-old woman. After enjoying sex for years, I find that my orgasm is harder to achieve and is not as intense as it once was. What can I do about this problem?

Between menopause (which usually happens at about age fifty-one) and the early sixties, estrogen supplies drift slowly downward. This affects, among other things, the quality of orgasm. Estrogen is a vasodilator and is therefore important to sexual arousal and lubrication. Ask your doctor about systemic HRT. If you don't want HRT, consider inserting an estradiol pellet, ring, or cream into your vagina often enough and at doses high enough to increase the thickness and water content of your vaginal lining (which your doctor can test for you). Many women find that, even hours after using estrogen cream, they become aroused and welcome sexual activity. The benefits of "estrogenization" of the perineal tissues, by the way, extends to the urethra, whose lining also atrophies in the absence of adequate amounts of estrogen; the results are stress incontinence (losing urine while coughing, laughing, or sneezing), a troublesome desire to urinate even when you've just been to the bathroom, and painful urination. Vaginal estrogen is also absorbed by the adjacent tissues around the urethra and can bring significant relief of these symptoms to an older patient.

My wife has been severely depressed for a year; recently she's improved enough to want to sleep with me again. The medicine she's taking for the blues (Prozac) has restored her interest in sex, but she finds it difficult and sometimes impossible to climax. What can we do?

Ask her doctor if her taking Actifed an hour before you go to bed together might relieve the problem, which is almost certainly due to her SSRI.

My doctor says testosterone will help maintain my muscle mass, restore my sense of energy and well-being, and improve my libido. She has measured my testosterone levels and found them very low. How will the testosterone be given to me?

Unfortunately but not surprisingly, most testosterone-replacement options have been developed for men. Only a few have been tested in women, and even fewer have been approved for use in the United States. Testosterone implants have been approved for postmenopausal women in Great Britain. Susan Davis, director of research at the Jean Hailes Foundation in South Clayton, Victoria, Australia, an expert in treating female sexual dysfunction, recommends an implant of 50 mg under the skin of the lower abdomen.[9] These implants have been used in postmenopausal Australian women; they enhance libido and improve bone density. The implant lasts from three to six months, but it is not approved for use in the United States. An oral preparation of estrogen and methyltestosterone is available, but methyltestosterone levels can't be measured by a blood test, so you and your doctor would have to judge when you've had an effect that's desirable or a side effect (like deepening voice or increased facial hair) that isn't. Besides masculinization, some other problems to watch for with testosterone treatment include a negative effect on serum lipids. Testosterone can lower the all-important high-density lipoprotein (HDL) or "good" cholesterol that protects women and men from developing coronary artery disease. *Before you take testosterone, make sure your doctor has measured your serum lipids and that your HDL is over 45 mg/dL.*

A transdermal patch is in development that will deliver testosterone (150 mcg per day) with a twice-weekly application. Transvaginal creams and gels that can be rubbed on the skin are also being developed.

Susan Davis reminds us that in some situations testosterone replacement is not a good idea. Moderate to severe acne will get worse, as will male pattern baldness in both sexes. Women who already have excess facial hair don't want more. Testosterone *must not be used* by pregnant women or women nursing babies.

I am seventy-two and am still interested in sex, but my husband died ten years ago. My friends think I'm ridiculous, but I'd like to have a partner.

You're not ridiculous. Women even more than men are capable of enjoying a richly satisfactory sex life into old age. Unfortunately, our culture assumes that women in general are not interested in sex for its own sake but only in the context of a loving (and monogamous) relationship. While that may be the ideal for both sexes, recreational sex is perfectly acceptable, and women are as capable as men of enjoying sex in the absence of romance. Another taboo I'd like to see erased is the idea that women can couple, marry, or sleep only with older men: physiologically, a seventy-two-year-old woman might find much more sexual satisfaction with a man a decade or more younger than she is than with a man her own age. Sexual exchanges that may not be ideal are certainly better than lives of enforced celibacy—and there is no reason to forgo them.

My husband likes to watch erotic videos as part of lovemaking. I think I ought to be enough to arouse him. Am I wrong?

Men respond to external cues like erotic pictures or films more than women do. It's not a rejection of you at all but may actually be an effort on his part to enhance your lovemaking.

My menstrual periods stopped six months ago, but I feel the same nausea and breast tenderness that I did with my pregnancies. I've been sexually active, but at fifty-three how can I be pregnant?

Even in the absence of menstrual periods for several months, it's entirely possible for an aging ovary to release a viable egg. You should be tested for the possibility of pregnancy—or for a possible tumor producing hormones that make you feel pregnant.

CHAPTER 11

The Lungs

IKE ALL THE other organ systems we've talked about, the lungs show gender specificity in function, mass, and susceptibility to disease. But unlike heart disease or depression, which have a distinctive array of symptoms depending on the patient's gender, the hallmark of lung disease is universal and eerily simple. The well-functioning lung does its job invisibly, a hushed whisper we mostly ignore; but when its function is compromised, we're helpless to do much else but struggle to breathe.

Every time I teach at the New York Presbyterian Hospital, my interns and residents ask me what pain or discomfort I think is the worst of all. Renal colic? Labor? A heart attack? All are terrible, I agree, but the worst suffering in my opinion is hunger for air. The medical word we use for it is *dyspnea* (literally, "difficult breath"). I still have trouble watching it. Patients who are the most short of breath speak in short phrases, eat slowly (because they can't breathe for the few seconds it takes to gulp down a mouthful of food), and have a characteristic, anxious—even terrified—expression as they struggle to move air in and out of their laboring chests.

Different diseases produce different kinds of dyspnea. The patterns and tone of each illness's labored breathing are so characteristic that I can sometimes make a diagnosis before entering the room. The patient with congestive heart failure, whose lungs are filling with fluid, is literally drowning; she breathes rapidly, but no matter how she tries, she doesn't have enough lung surface left to supply her with life-giving oxygen. The asthmatic doesn't have trouble getting air into his lungs, but blowing it out again takes enormous effort: the muscles of his air passages are in spasm, and he pushes air past the obstruction in a long, wheezing outward breath that seems to take forever. The patient with chronic obstructive lung disease—lungs stiff with secretions and scar tissue—leans forward, bracing his arms on a table, so that he is better positioned to blow to propel air out of his unyielding chest. Every exhalation has a characteristic whistling sound as the air passes the narrow hole he has made with his pursed lips to form a resistance against which he can blow. The anxious patient, on the edge of a panic attack, gasps, mouth wide open, with deep, unfettered breaths that come so rapidly, he grows dizzy and may actually faint.

And finally, one of the most affecting sights and sounds in all of those to which doctors are witness in the course of caring for patients: the deep gasping and isolated breaths called *agonal breathing* that signal that death is imminent. These breaths are spaced many seconds apart—perhaps no more than one in-and-out tremendous whoosh of air in five minutes, and they sound uncannily the same in all the dying. It is the last human activity we can see, and even though the heart and brain may mount an occasional surge of electrical activity for minutes and even hours after breathing stops, death—for all intents and purposes—has occurred. As an intern, I wondered if that whoosh was the sound of the soul leaving the body (although I never admitted this to my fellow interns, who seemed infinitely more worldly than I).

The breathing apparatus that evolved as life moved out of water to the shore is remarkable indeed. Masterfully fashioned, the lung filters out the harmful particles we breathe in, mounts a defense against those we cannot trap before they begin to do harm, helps maintain the proper chemical balance of the body, and finally delivers fresh, oxygen-rich air to the terminal, delicate sacs of its airways called the alveoli. These remarkable bubbles of tissue, only a single cell thick, abut the tiniest blood vessels of the pulmonary circulation, so that the used blood coming from our busily working tissues can surrender its burden of waste gas—carbon dioxide—and refuel with the oxygen we need for life. In 1628 William Harvey, the great English physiologist, recorded his tremendous discovery—that the blood travels in a great, closed circuit throughout the body—in a marvelous text, *De Motu Cordis* (Concerning the motion of the heart). He was the first to understand that the sole function of the heart is to collect blood from the body's cells, tissues, and organs and propel it along the veins into the right side of the heart, where it could be pumped through the blood vessels into the lungs, then be refreshed and purified and returned to the left side of the heart, only to be pumped forward once more and distributed throughout the body to supply it with life-giving oxygen. I think that in our intense concentration on the heart and the consequences of heart disease, doctors sometimes tend to forget the importance of the lungs, which in a sense the heart exists simply to serve.

WHAT'S THE DIFFERENCE BETWEEN MEN'S AND WOMEN'S LUNGS?

Women's lungs are smaller than those of men. Before you say "I knew it," I want to tell you something surprising: the lungs are smaller in women *even when we adjust for the smaller size of women's bodies.* Furthermore, women have lower levels of *hemoglobin,* the molecule in the blood that carries oxygen to tissues. Lower hemoglobin levels might seem to require *larger* lung volume, to compensate for the reduced amount of oxygen circulating through the lungs. But women's lungs are smaller, not larger, and we don't know why. Oddities like this can only serve as clues to the bigger picture that researchers have pursued for generations.

Long ago pulmonary physiologists figured out a few of the basic gender differences in normal lung function and constructed different tables of normal values for the tests doctors use to measure these functions. For example, women have less *residual volume* (the amount of air that remains in the lungs after expelling all the air possible in a single breath) and, predictably, a lower *vital capacity* (the amount of air that can be moved in and out of the lungs in a breath) than men. More recently researchers have discovered other gender-specific characteristics of the pulmonary system. Progesterone (the hormone that is more abundant after ovulation) stimulates breathing—perhaps an evolutionary adaptation to supply any newly fertilized egg with optimally oxygenated blood. Even lung efficiency is enhanced in midcycle, as oxygen and carbon dioxide diffuse more easily between the pulmonary capillaries and the alveolar sacs of the lung. As we discuss the lungs, let's take a critical look at a few diseases that have disproportionately severe or unusual symptoms in women: lung cancer, chronic obstructive pulmonary disease, asthma, pulmonary hypertension, and sleep apnea.

SMOKING: NOT AN EQUAL OPPORTUNITY KILLER!

Most women today would likely identify breast cancer as their most formidable enemy, but in 1987 lung cancer surpassed breast cancer as the chief malignancy killing American women. Between 1950 and 1995, the mortality rate from lung cancer increased by 500 percent among American females.[1] In 1999 in the United States 23,000 more women died from lung cancer than from breast cancer, and in 2000 the toll is expected to be 68,000: *more than 1.5 times as large as the toll from breast cancer*. Yet I have yet to see a ribbon of any color or a marathon run/walk organized by anyone to highlight the danger of smoking for women, or the need for more research on the particular susceptibility of women to nicotine addiction, or the outrageous vulnerability of women smokers to lung cancer, which is *three times* that of male smokers the same age! (My discussion here will focus on smoking-related lung cancer, but 20 to 30 percent of lung cancers occur in women who are nonsmokers; moreover, women get lung cancer at younger ages than men and are more likely to develop a more aggressive form.)

Why is the number of women smokers increasing? Why is their addiction more profound? Why are they so much more likely to develop tumors as a result of smoking—tumors that are distributed so differently in their lungs, compared to men's, that they are much harder to detect? I've asked Columbia University's deans repeatedly for permission to request money from tobacco companies for research on these and related issues. What better use for the enormous profits from an industry that continues to spread persuasive propaganda throughout the world, enticing more and more young people to begin a habit that causes one in every four cancer deaths in women?

Tobacco companies are in avid pursuit of the young female market. Their targeted marketing campaigns are especially effective on women, particularly teenage girls. Ads feature beautiful, strong young women—so distant from the tobacco user's reality, the increased risk for cancers of the mouth, pharynx, lung, colon, pancreas, kidney, and uterus, as well as coronary artery disease, stroke, and chronic lung disease. As one researcher has put it, "Smoking reduces the number of years that a woman can expect to live, no matter what her age."[2]

The peculiar and disproportionate interest that American females show in breast cancer seems to me to be another reflection of the emphasis our society puts on the value of women's reproductive capacity and sexual attractiveness. But if death were the primary issue, American women would be equally (if not more) obsessed with cardiovascular disease and with lung and colon cancer, all of which have higher mortality rates for women than for men. Recently at a health spa, a friend asked me to look at her (abnormal) exercise tolerance test; she had had a "silent" heart attack several years ago. In the course of the ensuing conversation, I reminded her that smoking was particularly deadly for her and warned her (not for the first time) that she must never put a cigarette in her mouth again. "I only have one in the evening with friends," she told me. I was dumbfounded—I had explained to her more than once that even one cigarette a day increases the risk for a heart attack. She told me she never even knew she had had a heart attack; that her physician had found the scar in a routine electrocardiogram done as part of the preparation for general anesthesia prior to surgery. Like most educated, health-conscious women, she had had an annual mammogram and Pap smear—but didn't know her HDL and LDL levels or that her high blood pressure increased her risk for coronary artery disease. I wondered how much counseling she had had from her doctors over the years not only about the risk factors for heart disease in women who smoke but about the deadly consequences of cigarettes (even that "one with a friend after dinner") for her lung health. She probably hadn't had much counseling about those things at all, which is a great shame. Convincing data demonstrate that smoking is a more important cause of coronary artery disease in women than in men: in fact, the life expectancy of women smokers in general is lower than that of men. It is the responsibility of physicians to educate their patients not only on the topics they want to hear about but also on the ones they do not.

At the beginning of the twentieth century, when "nice" women didn't smoke, men's rates of lung cancer far outstripped those of women. The Roaring Twenties ushered in an era of increasing pressure on women to smoke. During and after World War II, the increase in female smokers really began. Women took up smoking in huge numbers; more and more it became a mark of "equality" with men and of sophistication and "coolness" (as in the popular brand of cigarettes called Kools). Tobacco companies began to market specifically to women. To their everlasting shame, not only did they hide the fact of the tremendous addictiveness of nicotine, but as we now know, they deliberately enhanced the addictive properties of cigarettes to assure that the smoker would continue to indulge in the habit, even at the expense of health and of life itself.

The number of women smokers peaked in the 1960s, when one out of three women smoked. Foolishly, they believed they would not be subject to the same terrible consequences of smoking as men, because men had started smoking in meaningful numbers much earlier. But men also began to give it up sooner: in the mid-1950s, 55 percent of men smoked, but only 32 percent still smoked by 1993. In contrast, the number of female smokers began to taper off after the 1960s, and the decline caught up to that in men only in the early 1980s.

A crucial exception is the fact that today white adolescent girls are smoking in rapidly increasing numbers. (In contrast to white girls, the number of African American girl smokers is sharply decreasing; among high schoolers, the number was 32 percent lower in 1997 than in 1991!) By the age of fourteen, 15 percent of girls today are smoking, compared with only 9 percent of boys, although at the beginning of puberty (between the ages of ten and twelve), the number of those who smoke is identical (4 percent), which would indicate that more boys than girls stop smoking. And it is riskier for young girls to smoke: adolescent female smokers are more likely to retard their lung growth than young male smokers. Among teenage girls smoking shows signs of becoming an epidemic of staggering proportions. An important study of smoking in Canadian women tells us that there were 15.3 million women smokers in that country in 1997 and predicts that if fifteen-year-old Canadian adolescent girls continue to smoke, they will experience *51 percent of premature deaths among that population, outnumbering those who die of auto accidents, suicide, murder, and HIV/AIDS by fourteen to one!*[3]

Here are some facts to give your daughter and, if you smoke, to read every day:[4]

- *For the same number of cigarettes smoked, women have a 20 to 70 percent higher risk of developing lung cancer than men.* This is because they have more sensitivity to the cancer-causing substances in cigarettes.
- Most adult smokers begin using tobacco in adolescence; there are now more women smoking than men.
- The lag time between the appearance of lung cancer after smoking begins is about twenty years. This is why rates of this largely incurable malignancy have soared in women and now exceed those in men.
- When girls begin to smoke, they not only associate it with being cool and sophisticated but rapidly find that it keeps them thin (and that stopping it is associated with weight gain) and that it relieves feelings of anxiety and stress. By the time they are adults (between thirty and forty) and want to quit, *they are much less likely to be able to do so than men* of the same age and with a similar smoking history.
- The earlier smoking begins, the more likely it is to result in lung cancer, regardless of the number of cigarettes smoked per day or how deeply the patient inhales.
- Girls and women are more susceptible to tobacco advertising than males. In spite of this, a recent survey done by the Society for Women's Health Research of twenty-one women's magazines showed that while some (*New Woman, Self, Shape,* and *Weight*

Watchers) had no ads for cigarettes, three had three ads each (*McCall's, Glamour, Family Circle*), *Mademoiselle* had five, *Cosmopolitan* six, and *Vogue* nine. Nine other magazines carried from one to four ads for cigarettes.[5]

- Smoking is a cause of significant gum disease as well as tooth decay and, ultimately, tooth loss in patients over seventy. A study done in 1993 showed that almost 65 percent of men and 37 percent of women with the most extensive gum disease were previous tobacco users.[6]
- Smoking impairs fertility in women, increases menstrual problems, and produces premature menopause. Low-birth-weight babies born prematurely are one of the penalties paid for smoking during pregnancy.
- More than men, women use smoking to medicate depression and to control weight and anger.[7]
- One reason women find it harder than men to quit is that women are more likely to substitute food for their cigarette habit and become "supergainers" (gain more than twenty-five pounds after quitting) than men.

LUNG CANCER: IS IT THE SAME DISEASE IN WOMEN AS IN MEN?

Unfortunately, the consequences of smoking persist for a lifetime, and the younger people are when they started smoking, the higher the risk that they will develop lung cancer. This important fact has been publicized recently and has produced an explosion of requests for lung CAT scans, which will show an early (and much more curable) lesion than conventional X-rays. Women smokers are at even higher risk: although men have a higher incidence of central lesions, which occur in larger airways and produce symptoms earlier, women's lesions are more likely to be out in the periphery of the lung, where warning symptoms occur much later in the development of the cancer. It is reasonable for doctors to order a CAT scan for all smokers, but particularly for women who smoked early in adolescence and continued for several years before stopping.

Other recent news about women's unique susceptibility came from the *Journal of the National Cancer Institute* in December 2000, when investigators described the presence of a damaged gene (the K-ras gene) in women smokers with lung cancer that wasn't present in men with the disease. This genetic vulnerability, which cripples the body's ability to neutralize cancer-causing chemicals in smoke, is also the probable reason women are more vulnerable to damage from second-hand smoking than are men. The K-ras gene mutation is deadly; people who develop lung cancer with this lesion are four times more likely to die than patients without it. Without the defect, 70 percent of patients survive for five years. The K-ras mutation is found in 25 percent of a particular kind of lung cancer (an adenocarcinoma) almost exclusively found in smokers. Why the mutation makes women so vulnerable to malignancy is not really known, but scientists theorize that there are more receptors for estrogen on the surface of cells that have it. They think that the increased estrogen binding that results makes cells grow even more vigorously, eventually "crowding out" healthy cells with undamaged genes. This suggests that women ought to be tested for the K-ras mutation, just as they can be tested for the genetic mutations that are linked with breast and ovarian cancer (BRCA1 and BRCA2). Those who have the K-ras mutation could take tamoxifen, a hormone that blocks estrogen binding of defective cells. Certainly it makes one wonder if doctors should test women who have smoked for the mutation before they prescribe HRT postmenopausally, as the HRT might actually incite the production of cancerous cells.

A new case report supports the unique susceptibility of even young women smokers to unusual and virulent kinds of lung cancer. Most cancers of the lung are adenocarcinomas; the more rare kind, squamous cell pulmonary cancer (which usually develops after a long history of smoking), occurs in less than a third of malignancies in young people. In one reported case a squamous cell carcinoma appeared in a thirty-one-year-old woman, mother of one child, who had a history of intestinal cancer in her grandmother; she had been smoking seven cigarettes a day for fourteen years before her malignancy developed.[8] The cancer was particularly virulent, suggesting that the combination of genetic susceptibility and the more intense negative impact of smoking in females might have combined to produce this unusual event. The impact of pregnancy on the development and size (when discovered, the cancer was 12 by 10 cm—considered enormous) and the virulence of the tumor is also a factor to be taken into consideration. Unfortunately, the authors of the report did not mention whether they had tested the patient for genetic susceptibility, or whether her tumor was estrogen-receptor positive.

Cases like this one illustrate the urgent need for new techniques and testing modalities to identify women at particularly high risk for lung cancer. Michael Unger, the director of the Fox Chase Cancer Center's Pulmonary Cancer Detection and Prevention Program in Philadelphia, is doing just that; his center is emphasizing the importance of genetic vulnerability to this disease, which has a survival rate of only 14 percent compared with the 84 percent rate of breast cancer. Unger's group is working on a gene (CYP IAI) that is part of a family of genes that activate cancer-causing substances (carcinogens) in the body. They are studying a group of women with this high-risk gene to see if sophisticated detection techniques can identify early cancers in these patients and improve the survival of affected women.

Our society needs more information about the combination of factors that make even very young females who smoke vulnerable to these almost inevitably fatal tumors. Certainly lawyers would like to know about them—if a particular set of risk factors are known to make smoking more harmful to women as a group, they might have a better chance of bringing tobacco companies under control. At the very least, such young women would be better informed about the risks that smoking entails for them. That having been said, 20 to 30 percent of lung cancers occur in women who are nonsmokers; moreover, women get it at younger ages and are more likely to develop a more aggressive form than men.

CHRONIC OBSTRUCTIVE PULMONARY DISEASE

Chronic obstructive pulmonary disease (COPD) is another illness of the lungs that men and women experience differently. This incurable and persistent deterioration in lung function has several causes, only a few of which we understand. Cigarette smoking is one, and while deaths from COPD in women smokers continue to increase, the rates seem to have leveled off in men. Women smokers with this disease have more deteriorated lung function than men: the volume of air they can forcibly blow out in one second decreases more than that of men per *pack-year* (the number of packs smoked per day times the number of years they have smoked). Women smokers' airways are more likely to go into spasm and constrict than are those of men; a small consolation is that women with COPD respond better to the early use of oxygen, but they are less willing to accept the chronic use of oxygen than men.

In the developing world, the incidence of COPD is higher in females than males, probably because of females' greater exposure to indoor air pollution from cooking and heating oils—and to tobacco smoke from men's cigarettes. In the United States, men and women are equally affected. COPD is least frequent in countries with the lowest smoking rates.

As is the case with so many illnesses, there is gender prejudice in the diagnosis of this disease. Doctors are less likely to make the diagnosis in women than they are in men. A 2001 study by Kenneth R. Chapman and his associates of the Asthma Center and Pulmonary Rehabilitation Program at Toronto Western Hospital showed that when doctors were presented with hypothetical cases of patients with identical symptoms, the same smoking histories, and the same abnormalities in lung function tests, they correctly diagnosed 64 percent of male patients but only 49 percent of female patients with COPD![9] Chapman commented that doctors are unlikely to order basic studies of pulmonary function even when confronted with a patient who is short of breath, wheezes, and has a history of heavy smoking: only 22 percent in this test said they would order such testing, and they were much more likely to pursue an evaluation of cardiac rather than lung function.

One of the mysteries about COPD is that only 15 percent of smokers develop the disease. Its actual cause is still being debated. The "Dutch hypothesis" implicates a tendency of airways to be "hyperreactive" and constrict in response to noxious stimuli; the "British hypothesis" holds that a tendency to secrete large amounts of mucus from glands in the tissues of the airways is the responsible agent. The most intriguing idea, though, is that the airways are overwhelmed by destructive proteins (called proteases and cathepsins) that are secreted by inflammatory cells. Some patients are vulnerable to these destructive proteins because they lack an essential chemical, alpha 1-antitrypsin, which destroys them. Moreover, cigarette smoke is a potent inhibitor of alpha 1-antitrypsin, so that patients who lack adequate amounts of the defending protein to begin with may be particularly vulnerable to cigarette smoking.

ASTHMA

Asthma is an illness in which the air passages that carry oxygen into the lungs are chronically inflamed and are narrowed by spasm of the muscles that control their diameter. Though it is sometimes thought of as more common in females, asthma affects many more boys during childhood, at earlier ages than girls. Boys can have a first attack as young as three, while the disease becomes apparent in girls at about age eight. The main reason is that boys have smaller airways, relative to the volume of their lungs, than girls, and as a result, they have lower rates of air flow. (For those of you who are parents and smoke, it's important to know that secondhand smoke causes bronchospasm in infants. This can be more of a problem for male infants than for females, but it's extremely important that babies not be exposed to any secondhand smoke, no matter what their gender!) During adolescence, usually at about the time of puberty, the pattern of asthma occurrence shifts, and from ages fifteen through forty-nine, females have more asthma than males.

More than 14.6 million Americans suffer from asthma, which ranks sixth among our chronic diseases. Inexplicably and alarmingly, between 1982 and 1992, it increased 82 percent in females, compared with only a 29 percent increase in men! Even more sobering, the death rate for women increased 59 percent, compared with a 34 percent increase in men. Clearly more study needs to be given to the causes and complications of asthma in women. What we do understand fairly well is what we have come to expect when we take a closer look at many diseases: that hormones are standing in the wings, playing a shadowy role.

Hormones have a particularly noticeable effect on the severity and timing of asthma attacks, a discovery that can improve an asthmatic's life considerably. One study showed that asthmatic women near the beginning of the menstrual cycle had four times as many emergency room visits as other asthmatic women. The lower concentration of estrogen in women during the period immediately before menstruation unquestionably affects drug metabolism, and the bronchodilators women use are more rapidly processed by the liver—and thus are less effective—premenstrually than at any other time. In fact, almost half (46 percent) of emergency room visits by asthmatic women are in the perimenstrual interval (day 26–4 of the menstrual cycle).* Oral contraceptives can eliminate this problem for such women, by stabilizing hormone levels across the cycle.[10] The number of cytokines (proteins released by cells), which play a major role in inflaming airways, increases at the time of menses; the oral contraceptive pill also eliminates this phenomenon.

When I explain all this to my asthmatic women patients for the first time, they often say to me, with tears in their eyes, "At last! Now I can tell my doctor I'm not crazy when I tell him that if I'm going to have an asthma attack, it's always just before I menstruate!" (At least one unfortunate opinion has it that all women with premenstrual asthma are probably under the influence of premenstrual tension, which is said to be the actual reason for their symptoms.[11] It's very important for doctors to distinguish between the diagnosis of asthma and the blanket diagnosis of PMS. I hope it is clear by now that hard evidence supports the cyclical variations of symptoms and illnesses in women.)

In general, patients with severe asthma have more trouble during pregnancy, particularly during the end of the second trimester. This is

---

* Day 26 of the month preceding menses and the first 4 days of the next month.

the time in pregnancy when total blood volume is highest, and the demands on the heart are maximal; symptoms improve in the last months of gestation and within three months of the baby's birth return to a prepregnancy pattern and intensity. If asthma isn't well controlled during pregnancy, the baby tends to have a lower-than-normal birth weight. The safety of asthmatic medication during pregnancy has been fairly well documented: in general steroids should be avoided, but bronchodilators like albuterol haven't been demonstrated to be harmful in humans, and terbutaline has been shown to be safe in humans. If a pregnant asthmatic needs antibiotics, then penicillins, cephalosporins, and erythromycin have all proven safe to use. Tetracycline, on the other hand, should *not* be used, as it creates tooth and bone malformations in the fetus.

Another gender-specific feature of asthma is the greater sensitivity of women's airways to endotoxin, a substance produced by bacteria that is abundant in dust, particularly agricultural dust. Even nonallergic and nonasthmatic people can have very severe airway spasm in response to inhaling endotoxin; this troublesome response to the poison, which when inhaled apparently mobilizes inflammatory cells in the lungs, may have a genetic basis. These cells release cytokines, which in turn attract more inflammatory cells; a vicious cycle is set up in the susceptible person. In 1999 David A. Schwartz of the University of Iowa studied this phenomenon, reporting in the *American Journal of Respiratory and Critical Care Medicine* that seven of the eight people who reacted most violently to endotoxin inhalation were women; this is reasonable, given what we know about women's superior ability to mount an *inflammatory response* to challenges by infective agents compared with men.

Do Asthmatic Men and Women Have Different Symptoms?

There are several differences in the way men and women experience asthma. Women are much more likely to be smokers and to have more severe disease (measured by difficulty breathing in the morning and during sleep, and by the number of admissions to an intensive care unit) than men. One Canadian expert, Ian Mitchell of Alberta Children's Hospital in Calgary, has said he believes women have a more chronic form of the disease, while men's attacks deteriorate into crises more quickly. Another study supported this idea: in a population of patients admitted to an emergency room with asthma attacks, men had worse results from tests for pulmonary function, but women were more likely to be admitted to the hospital and to have another attack within two weeks after discharge.[12] Mitchell pointed out that these differences in the clinical course of an attack might be due to differences in the way men and women metabolize the drugs used for treating the illness; he urged that physicians be more aggressive with their female patients. Moreover, different things may trigger attacks in women, of which both doctors and patients should be aware. Women report a history of more hay fever and other allergies than men, and their attacks more commonly have psychosocial causes (62 percent of women, compared with 49 percent of men)

Johns Hopkins's Jerry Krishnan warns that being an African American woman may result in less adequate care for asthma. In a study of over 5,000 patients, treatment differences were striking: blacks were less likely than whites to use inhaled steroids, have enough information to manage their own attacks, know how to avoid asthma triggers, and see specialists. African American women were less likely to use their medications as prescribed and saw specialists less frequently than men.[13]

PRIMARY PULMONARY HYPERTENSION

In the mysterious disease known as primary pulmonary hypertension (PPH), which occurs almost exclusively in young and middle-age women, the pulmonary blood vessels constrict, causing the right side of the heart to pump blood through the lung with much more effort, essentially raising the blood pressure in the lungs. The cause may be a defect in the cells that line the blood vessels (the endothelial cells), which no longer can maintain a balance in the substances they produce to dilate and constrict the pulmonary blood vessels.

James E. Loyd and his colleagues at Vanderbilt University Medical

Center have given us an important lead in understanding the causes of PPH: they've discovered that a defective gene (like the K-ras gene associated with lung cancer) may be responsible. In normal people, this gene (bone morphogenic protein receptor two, or BMPR2) controls the proliferation of cells in the lungs' blood vessels and prevents them from exuberant and disorderly growth. When the gene is defective, cell multiplication spirals out of control and plugs up the openings of blood vessels in the lungs.

One of the most striking differences in PPH between men and women is the response to medications used to cut appetite. One study found that women who used an appetite depressant called aminorex fumarate were four times more likely than men to develop PPH. Fifty percent of those women died. In 1996 fenfluramine began to be prescribed in Canada to control appetite; many patients also received another medication, phentermine, to bolster the effect of the fenfluramine; the combination was called *fen-phen*. In 1998 doctors wrote 18 million prescriptions for fen-phen in the United States alone! Women who took the combination for longer than three months had a 23 percent increase in the occurrence of PPH, which also produced valvular heart disease in some patients. Both conditions were much more frequent in women than in men; 30 percent of women on the combination developed one or both disorders.

The diagnosis of PPH can be difficult for doctors to make, because the early symptom is shortness of breath upon exertion, which doctors often attribute to lack of physical fitness. I have a patient who determinedly worked out on a treadmill every day, forcing herself to do so in spite of increasing breathlessness, because her physicians told her she was simply "out of shape." When the disease is well advanced, the right side of the heart simply can't meet the challenge of mounting pressures in the lungs and dilates. Blood flows backward as well as forward with each beat, causing the veins of the neck to become distended, a telltale sign of serious PPH. It's important to note that 10 to 20 percent of patients with sleep apnea (disturbances in normal sleep, which I will discuss in a moment) have PPH.

One final warning about PPH. High blood pressure in the lungs isn't just a problem for adults. Women who take aspirin and non-steroidal anti-inflammatory drugs like ibuprofen during pregnancy are *twenty-one times more likely* to have a baby with PPH. One thousand to two thousand babies a year are born with the disorder. Fortunately, this is a preventable disease.

SLEEP APNEA: NOT JUST A PROBLEM FOR MEN

Obstructive sleep apnea is, unfortunately, another example of a disease that is chronically underdiagnosed in women. In sleep apnea, breathing stops periodically for ten seconds or longer during sleep; the patient usually awakens with a loud snort as she resumes breathing. The disorder wreaks havoc on the patient's nervous system, heart, and lungs. It is almost always found in very overweight patients, who awaken so often that rest is disturbed and they are exhausted during waking hours. Because of the chronic fatigue that these people experience, they are more prone to accidents than the normal population. Until quite recently, doctors thought sleep apnea was a predominantly (eight to one) male disorder, but a study of diagnosing the disease in obese women who were attending a clinic for eating disorders proved that it is much more common in females than that: the actual incidence ratio is only two or three males to one female. Nevertheless, the misperception lingers, and doctors often overlook the diagnosis in women

CYSTIC FIBROSIS

When I was a medical student, one of my most memorable patients, Conrad, was a charming young man who was dying of cystic fibrosis. I can still see him, half the size of a normal twenty-year-old, straining to cough up the thick, viscous mucus that was suffocating him. We had no idea at that time what caused the disease, but it is due to a combination of cell defects (one of which is a defect in the channel in the cell membrane that controls chloride concentrations in sweat) in the skin, lungs, and other organs, including the pancreas. In 1989 scientists cloned the specific gene (which is located on chromosome 7 in humans) responsible for the disease.

The kind of defect in the responsible gene determines which of the patient's organs will be most affected. Most patients, like Conrad, die of lung failure; an abundance of thick, tenacious mucus plugs up their airways, making them vulnerable to infection and inflammation of lung tissue. Others die of pancreatic failure or intestinal obstruction. (The most ruinous assault of the disease is on the intestinal tract.)

The course of the disease has many differences between males and females; if researchers could make sense of them, we would have important clues about how the disease works. For example, we might better understand what makes patients die sooner rather than later, and what protects some organs from the ravages of the illness and destroys others. While most patients die of lung problems, others die of pancreatic failure.

One unexplained gender difference in patients with cystic fibrosis is that men generally live longer (their median life expectancy is thirty-three years) than women (twenty-nine years). While patients with the lowest weights for their heights die sooner, affected girls have better weights for the heights they achieve, even though they have poorer caloric intake and higher resting energy expenditure. This isn't accounted for by excluding the girls who die from the most serious forms of the illness. Although recent animal studies show that estrogen and progesterone may change the function of the cell's chloride channels, we have no data yet about their impact in humans. In any case, the importance of the role of hormones in female vulnerability is belied by the fact that the risk of death for girls increases steadily after the first year of life up to age twenty, after which survival patterns are similar between the two sexes. We also know that girls' pulmonary function deteriorates more rapidly than that of boys throughout the course of the illness. Why is this so? At least part of the answer is girls' particular and unexplained sensitivity to a bacterium that typically colonizes the lung in cystic fibrosis, *Pseudomonas aeruginosa*. Girls are infected earlier than boys (before their eighth year, compared with 8.6 years of age in boys) and they acquire a more virulent form earlier (10 versus 11.5 years of age) than boys. Differences in fitness, which has an important impact on survival, may be part of the answer too: girls had a much worse exercise performance than boys, although this was generally because their lung function deteriorates more quickly over the course of the disease.

If we could learn why men with cystic fibrosis live on average about four years longer than women, we would have a valuable insight into how to prevent and treat the disease. Like all diseases that affect males and females differently, cystic fibrosis is a compelling example of the fact that tracing the gender *differences* in the way people experience illness makes researchers ask questions they never would otherwise have asked, questions that lead them to valuable discoveries. In this case, it would be particularly valuable to unravel the secret of boys' advantage over girls. In a life that ends before thirty, four years would be a real gift.

WHAT DOES THE NEW SCIENCE MEAN FOR YOU?

Like many women, I smoke "light" cigarettes. Are these safer than other kinds of cigarettes?

More women than men smoke "lights": in the European Union, 48 percent of women smokers choose them, while only 32 percent of men do so. The difference increases with age: in the group at most risk for lung cancer (forty-five to sixty-four years old), 60 percent of women smoke "lights," but the number of men who do so stays at about 33 percent.

Initially low-tar/nicotine cigarettes appeared to lower the risk of cancer for those who used them, but when the data were corrected for *the number of cigarettes smoked daily,* the advantage disappeared. People who choose low-tar/nicotine cigarettes may be more cautious about smoking unrestrainedly than others—the real reason for their relatively lower risk for cancer.

A recent increase in a previously rare form of lung cancer has been linked to smoking "lights"; this cancer occurs deep in the lungs and is thought to be due to what the tobacco industry calls "smoker compensation": the person inhales the smoke more deeply, to prolong nicotine absorption time from a cigarette that contains lower levels of the drug.

My husband and I want to stop smoking. How can we accomplish it?

You probably have different reasons for wanting to kick the habit: in a survey of 1,000 smokers,[14] the commonest reason men wanted to quit was to improve their sex lives; the second was shortness of breath. Women wanted most to improve their health and that of their family and to preserve their appearance.

Your husband is more likely than you to want to quit cold turkey (42 percent of men versus 30 percent of women); you'll be more interested in asking your doctor for cessation products (58 percent versus 45 percent). This may be because men are less willing to visit the doctor in the first place: when nicotine-replacement therapy changed from prescription to over the counter, the sales in France doubled within two months.[15] Notwithstanding, nicotine-replacement therapy is less successful in women than in men; antidepressants may be more effective to help females kick the habit than nicotine patches or gum.

You'll have more intense withdrawal symptoms than your husband: you'll experience more stress, irritability, weight gain, depression, and anxiety. If you do gain a significant amount of weight (nicotine actually speeds up your metabolism), you'll be more likely to return to smoking. In some important respects, the rewards are greater for women than for men who stop smoking: women who smoke have almost double the risk of myocardial infarction and for developing lung cancer than men; the risk for a heart attack is even higher if smoking is combined with oral contraceptives.

Can my pregnant wife go scuba diving with me?

Sex probably doesn't affect an individual's ability to scuba dive: although women have smaller lungs than men, more body fat, and less upper body strength and use less air per minute, these facts aren't very important in recreational diving. Pregnancy, though, is a special situation, and animal studies have shown a higher incidence of fetal abnormalities as a consequence of decompression sickness. If a pregnant diver does develop a gas embolism, she'll need hyperbaric therapy, which poses a risk to her unborn child; the fetal eye is vulnerable to high concentrations of oxygen.

Pregnant women who dive should stay in water no deeper than thirty-three feet to avoid decompression sickness. Nausea, gastroesophageal reflux, and discomfort from a large abdomen may make diving uncomfortable. There is no evidence that diving has a negative effect in very early pregnancies.

My husband and I are moving to Los Angeles. Is our risk for lung cancer from air pollution different?

Researchers W. Lawrence Beeson and his colleagues at Loma Linda University in California studied more than 4,000 female and 2,000 male, white nonsmoking volunteers over a fifteen-year period and found that 20 of those women and 16 men were diagnosed with lung cancer.[16] A careful analysis of possible provocative agents in those patients showed that both sexes, when exposed to increased levels of sulfur dioxide, had an increased risk of lung cancer, but only men exposed to high ozone levels (80 parts per billion [ppb; the Environmental Protection Agency says the upper limit of ozone that's tolerable is 120 ppb]) had three times as much risk for lung cancer as men who were not similarly exposed. Women did not show the same vulnerability to high ozone levels; doctors speculated that this might be due to men's greater exposure to the outdoors than women's. Others suggested that estrogen might have a protective effect on women's lungs that makes them less vulnerable to air pollution. I'm not convinced that either explanation is the whole or even part of the story about why men seem to be more vulnerable to smog-filled air than women.

My husband insists on smoking around our new twins, a boy and a girl. Will their health be affected?

Your son is more likely to develop asthma as a result of your husband's habit than your daughter, but both run an increased risk of respiratory illnesses, including colds, bronchitis, and pneumonia, if they are exposed to secondhand smoke; even pets have an increased risk for pulmonary disease in a house where someone smokes.

I stopped smoking twenty years ago, but before that I smoked three packs a day for twenty years. Am I still at risk for lung or heart disease?

In women, the risk for a heart attack drops substantially by the first year or two, then decreases more gradually until ten to fifteen or more years after stopping.

Women like Demi Moore and Madonna are espousing cigar smoking as chic. Are cigars less dangerous than cigarettes?

Cigars are not a safer choice than cigarettes; the risk for death related to smoking is the same. But cigars work a little differently: because the smoke is less acidic than that of cigarettes, nicotine can be absorbed within the oral cavity. In fact, nicotine absorption goes on even if the cigar is unlit, but just held in the mouth!

I've just come back from a seventeen-hour plane trip from Japan. Last night I woke up with a knifelike pain in my chest, and I've been very short of breath. What should I do?

Being confined for hours to a narrow airplane seat without enough room or opportunity to stretch can cause a blood clot in the veins of your legs (called thrombophlebitis). This condition may not be terribly painful, but a piece of the clot can break off and land in the right side of the heart, where it is pumped out into the lungs and lodges in one of the blood vessels there, preventing enough blood from reaching that section of the lung. The affected lung tissue dies and causes an irritation of the transparent thin sac of tissue covering the lung (the pleura). Moving the lung against the inflamed pleura during the course of breathing causes a characteristic, knifelike pain that signals a problem.

Women who are on oral contraceptives or who are pregnant are at increased risk for this to happen, because estrogen makes the blood more coaguable.

You'll need a magnetic resonance angiogram (MRA) of your chest to show whether you've actually blocked off a part of the pulmonary circulation with a clot, causing the death of the tissue beyond the site. If that's the case, your doctor will give you a blood-thinning medication and keep you on it for at least three months. If you continue the anticoagulation for a year, then discontinue it, the likelihood of this happening again is the same as if you stopped after three months: 5 percent.

To make sure that you are not at higher-than-normal risk for clotting, your doctor will order special tests, including one test for a mutation in the gene that makes prothrombin, one of the components of the clotting mechanism. If you do have a fundamental abnormality, you may have to decide whether to agree to lifelong anticoagulation in view of the risk of bleeding; to make sure the amount of anticoagulant medication you're taking is adequate, you'll have to bear the annoyance of needing periodic monitoring blood examinations.

You'll also have to stop taking the pill, which is known to increase the chances to develop clots, so you'll need another method of birth control.

My father has been a smoker for years, and has been increasingly incapacitated by a cough and shortness of breath. Lately he's been nodding off to sleep, and his feet and legs are very swollen. Is there a connection here, and what should I do about it?

Your father has such advanced chronic obstructive pulmonary disease (COPD) that he is no longer able to get enough oxygen to his tissues. Inflammation and scarring have so damaged the architecture of his lungs that he is perfusing with blood areas of his lungs that don't get properly aerated. Other areas of his lungs may be getting air into them, but there is so much destruction in his lungs that these areas are not near any blood vessels, so proper gas exchange (which depends on removing carbon dioxide from blood in the lungs and resaturating it with life-giving oxygen) is no longer possible. As a result, his skin is a dusky purple (because of lack of oxygen in his tissues), and he is nodding off to sleep because the amount of carbon dioxide in the blood supplying his brain has so increased. In fact, he's been this way so long that his impulse to take a breath is no longer driven by the level of carbon dioxide in his blood, but by the *lack of adequate amounts of oxygen* in his tissues (hypoxia). High levels of CO_2 in the blood are sedating, which is why your dad spends most of his time asleep (CO_2 narcosis).

Why are his feet swelling? Because the acid-base balance of his body has become tremendously shifted to the acid side, and he no longer has adequate amounts of oxygen in his blood; a high concentration of acid in the blood coupled with a lower-than-normal oxygen level raises the pressure in the pulmonary circulation so high that he has pulmonary hypertension or high blood pressure in his lungs. The right side of the heart has become overwhelmed with the task of moving blood into the lungs against this tremendously increased resistance and goes into failure: it can no longer pump out all the blood delivered to it, and the pressure in the veins that has built up as a result causes fluid (edema) to collect in his tissues, particularly in the dependent portions of his body like his feet and legs. Your father's illness is called *cor pulmonale,* heart disease secondary to lung disease.

Cor pulmonale is much more common in men than in women *except in societies in which women cook indoors using fuel like coal in their ovens.* In these countries, women not only have earlier and more severe chronic lung disease, but they are more likely than men to develop right heart failure and do so fifteen years earlier than men.

Cor pulmonale patients used to be considered untreatable and once went on to die. They were literally wheeled to the back of the ward, where they made no fuss (because they were always sedated as a result of their own illness) and eventually slept themselves to death, as it were. In the 1950s and 1960s doctors at Columbia University College of Physicians and Surgeons (led by M. Irené Ferrer and Rejane M. Harvey, two rare women scientist-physicians who made critically important contributions to cardiovascular and pulmonary medicine in an era when most women never even reached a medical laboratory) were able to define the disturbances in right heart pressure and the pressures in the diseased lung very precisely by using the then-new cardiac catheter. These women proved that in these patients right heart failure could be corrected by a combination of vigorous attention to improving their lung function and by using the same cardiac medications used to treat other types of heart failure: digitalis and diuretics (water pills). Cor pulmonale became a reversible disease. Patients with chronic obstructive pulmonary disease were taught to use a combination of mechanical ventilatory aids and antibiotics when necessary that greatly improved their condition.

Even advanced lung disease can be helped. If you are becoming increasingly short of breath, particularly if you have smoked for many years, ask your doctor to test your lung function, *remembering that the diagnosis of COPD is made correctly less often in women than in men.* The earlier the reason for your shortness of breath is discovered, the easier it will be to treat it, slow down its progress, and even eliminate it.

Coda

EVEN THOUGH THIS book is filled with hundreds of facts about the differences between men and women, it is only a beginning. In five years I'll have to write another one, infinitely more sophisticated and replete with the answers to questions we've only begun to formulate.

In a very real sense, the new gender-specific science is a gift of women to the whole human family. It is women, after all, who challenged the scientific establishment's policy of doing research only on men, who reminded it that their own experience of their bodies was different from what scientists believed it to be, and who pointed out that when doctors assumed that they could treat women as though they were merely small men, they made a tremendous intellectual gaffe.

Using gender as a unique prism through which to view and better understand normal human function and the experience of disease is one of the most important new ideas in medicine. Everywhere researchers look for differences between men and women, they find them. And every time they find a new one, it prompts questions they never would otherwise have even thought to ask. The new knowledge about women is forcing a correction and expansion of male models of normal human function and the workings of illness to impair and destroy it. Inevitably, doctors will use the new knowledge to revise their ideas of how to prevent and to cure disease. The current emphasis on women's health, which often—regrettably—does not include a comparison of information about females and males, will morph into a newer, broader discipline: that of gender-specific medicine. No certifying examinations will qualify a doctor as a "specialist in women's health"; rather, doctors will all be trained in the unique features of both men's and women's biology and in the ways sex modifies the signs and symptoms of illness. All doctors will be gender-specific doctors, who treat men and women more accurately and more effectively, and who above all are more cognizant of the complexity of what it means to be a male or a female.

Wanting to learn more about women and contrast it to our knowledge of men is not a matter of political correctness or a product of feminist angst. It is an intellectual imperative. Correctly used, the natural experiment of biological sex is one of the most powerful tools we have been given to help us understand the human condition. Eve's apple, as I read the old tale, was the ultimate prize that Paradise had to offer.

Notes

CHAPTER I: Eve's Question: "How Am I Different from Adam?"

1. Marianne Legato, M.D., and Carol Colman, *The Female Heart: The Truth About Women and Coronary Artery Disease* (New York: Simon and Schuster, 1991), p. 252.

2. Anna C. Mastroianni, Ruth Faden, and Daniel Federman, eds., Committee on the Ethical and Legal Issues Relating to the Inclusion of Women in Clinical Studies, Division of Health Sciences Policy, Institute of Medicine, *Women and Health Research: Ethical and Legal Issues of Including Women in Clinical Studies,* vol. 1 (Washington, D.C.: National Academy Press, 1994).

3. R. R. Faden and T. L. Beauchamp, *A History and Theory of Informed Consent* (New York: Oxford University Press, 1986).

4. P.L.93–348.

5. National Institutes of Health, Office of Human Subjects Research, "NIH Policies and Procedures for Protecting Human Subjects: The NIH Multiple Project Assurance (MPA)," revised March 2, 1995 (Bethesda, Md.: National Institutes of Health); online at http://ohsr.od.nih.gov/guidelines.php3part3.

6. U.S. Department of Health and Human Services, *Women's Health: Report of the Public Health Service Task Force on Women's Health Issues,* 2 vols. (1985).

7. U.S. House of Representatives, Committee on Energy and Commerce, Subcommittee on Health and the Environment, testimony of Mark V. Nadel on problems in implementing the National Institutes of Health policy on women in study populations, June 18, 1990 (Washington, D.C.: General Accounting Office).

8. National Institutes of Health, National Commission for the Protection of Human Subjects of Biomedical and Behavioral Research, *The Belmont Report: Ethical Principles and Guidelines for the Protection of Human Subjects,* April 18, 1979; online at http://ohsr.od.nih.gov/mpa/belmont.php3.

CHAPTER 2: The Brain

1. E. Nagy, K. A. Loveland, H. Orvos, and P. Molnar, "Gender-Related Physiologic Differences in Human Neonates and the Greater Vulnerability of Males to Developmental Brain Disorders," *Journal of Gender-Specific Medicine* 4(2001):41–49.
2. Committee on Understanding the Biology of Sex and Gender Differences, *Exploring the Biological Contributions to Human Health: Does Sex Matter?* (Washington, D.C.: National Academy Press, 2001); online at http://www.nap.edu/catalog/10028.html.
3. G. Grön, A. P. Wunderlich, M. Spitzer, et al., "Brain Activation During Human Navigation: Gender Different Neural Networks as Substrate of Performance," *Nature Neuroscience* 3(2000):404–8.
4. B. R. Ott, W. C. Heindel, Z. Tan, and R. B. Noto, "Lateralized Cortical Perfusion in Women with Alzheimer's Disease," *Journal of Gender-Specific Medicine* 3(2000):29–35.

CHAPTER 3: Drug Metabolism

1. M. L. Chen et al., "Pharmacokinetic Analysis of Bioequivalence Trials: Implications for Sex-Related Issues in Clinical Pharmacology and Biopharmaceutics," *Clinical Pharmacology and Therapeutics* 68(2000):510.
2. J. B. Schwartz, "The Evaluation of Pharmacologic Therapy in Humans: A Brief Summary of the Drug Evaluation Process and Guidelines for Clinical Trials as They Relate to Women," *Journal of Gender-Specific Medicine* 4(2001).

CHAPTER 4: The Gastrointestinal Tract

1. C. Hawkey et al., "NSAIDs; Men Are from Mars, Women Are from Venus: Sex-Related Differences in Ulcer Disease Expression and the Influence of *Helicobacter pylori,*" *Gut* 42, Suppl. 1(1998):T13.
2. M. Matsui et al., "The Prognosis of Patients with Gastric Cancer Possessing Sex Hormone Receptors," *Surgery Today* 22(1992):421.
3. Michael D. Gershon, *The Second Brain: The Scientific Basis of Gut Instinct and*

a Groundbreaking New Understanding of Nervous Disorders of the Stomach and Intestine (New York: HarperPerennial Library, 1998).

4. D. A. Drossman, "Irritable Bowel Syndrome: A Multifactorial Disorder," *Hospital Practice* 23(1988):119–33.

5. F. Lonnqvist, L. Nordfors, and M. Schalling, "Leptin and Its Potential Role in Human Obesity," *Journal of Internal Medicine* 245(1999):643–52.

6. R. Kaltiala-Hein, A. Rissanen, M. Rimpela, and P. Rantanene, "Bulimia and Bulimic Behaviour in Middle Adolescence: More Common Than Thought?" *Acta Psychiatrica Scandinavica* 100(1999):33–39.

7. D. Herzog, J. Bradburn, and K. Newman, "Sexuality in Males with Eating Disorders," in A. E. Anderson, ed., *Practical Comprehensive Treatment of Anorexia Nervosa and Bulimia* (New York: Bruner/Mazel, 1990), 40–53.

8. A. E. Anderson, T. Gray, and J. Holman, "Osteopenia in Males with Eating Disorders," paper presented at the Seventh International Conference on Eating Disorders, New York, 1996.

CHAPTER 5: The Heart and Circulatory System

1. J. M. Tobin et al., "Sex Bias in Considering Coronary Bypass Surgery," *Annals of Internal Medicine* 107(1987):19.

2. S. G. Haynes and M. Feinleib, "Women, Work and Coronary Heart Disease: Prospective Findings from the Framingham Heart Study," *American Journal of Public Health* 70(1980):133–41.

3. M. Frankenhaeusen, "The Psychophysiology of Workload Stress and Health: Comparison Between the Sexes," *Annals of Behavioral Medicine* 12(1991):197.

4. K. A. Schulman et al., "The Effect of Race and Sex on Physicians' Recommendations for Cardiac Catheterizations," *New England Journal of Medicine* 340(1999):618.

5. American Medical Association, Council on Ethical and Judicial Affairs, "Gender Disparities in Clinical Decision Making," *Journal of the American Medical Association* 266(1991):559.

CHAPTER 6: The Immune System

1. A. M. Silverstine and N. R. Rose, "There Is Only One Immune System! The View from Immunopathology," *Seminars in Immunology* 12(2000):173.

2. R. G. Lahita, "The Role of Sex Hormones in Systemic Lupus Erythematosus," *Current Opinion in Rheumatology* 11(5) (1999):352–56.

3. R. D. Inman et al., "Systemic Lupus Erythematosus in Men: Genetic and Endocrine Features," *Archives of Internal Medicine*: 142(1982):1813–15.

4. M. D. Lockshin, "Biology and Gender: Why Do Women Have Rheumatic Disease?" *Scandinavian Journal of Rheumatology* 27, Suppl. 107(1998):5–9.

5. M. Nikezic-Ardolic et al., "Gender Differences in Cellular Response," *Lupus* 8(1999):375–79.

6. M. D. Lockshin et al., "Gender, Biology and Human Disease: Report of a Conference," *Lupus* 8(1999):335.

7. M. Zuk and K. A. McKean, "Sex Differences in Parasitic Infections: Patterns and Processes," *International Journal for Parasitology* 26(1996):1009–18.

8. N. Diagne et al., "Increased Susceptibility to Malaria During the Early Postpartum Period," *New England Journal of Medicine* 343(2000):598–603.

9. E. M. Long et al., "Gender Differences in HIV-1 Diversity at Time of Infection," *Nature Medicine* 6(2000):71–75.

10. R. M. Greenblatt, "Impact of the Ovulatory Cycle on Virologic and Immunologic Markers in HIV Infected Women," *Journal of Infectious Diseases* 181(2000):82–90.

11. J. K. Kiecolt-Glaser et al., "Negative Behavior During Marital Conflict Is Associated with Immunological Down-Regulation," *Psychosomatic Medicine* 55(1993): 395–409.

CHAPTER 7: The Skeleton

1. B. L. Riggs et al., "The Assembly of the Adult Skeleton During Growth and Maturation: Implications for Senile Osteoporosis," *Journal of Clinical Investigation* 104(1999):671–72.

2. J. P. Bilezikian et al., "Increased Bone Mass as a Result of Estrogen Therapy in a Man with Aromatase Deficiency," *New England Journal of Medicine* 339(1998):599–603.

3. C. Gomez et al., "Vitamin D Receptor Gene Polymorphisms, Bone Mass, Bone Loss and Prevalence of Vertebral Fracture: Differences in Postmenopausal Women and Men," *Osteoporosis International* 10(1999):175–82.

4. E. Barrett-Connor et al., "Low Levels of Estradiol Are Associated with Vertebral Fractures in Older Men, but Not Women: The Rancho Bernardo Study," *Journal of Clinical Endocrinology and Metabolism* 85(2000):219–23.

5. J. P. Bilezikian, "Gender Specificity and Osteoporosis," *Journal of Gender-Specific Medicine* 3(2000):6.

6. J. P. Bilezikian, "Commentary: Osteoporosis in Men," *Journal of Clinical Endocrinology and Metabolism* 84(1999):3431–34.

7. F. Iqbal et al., "Declining Bone Mass in Men with Chronic Pulmonary Disease," *Chest* 116(1999):1616–24.

8. A. P. Toth and F. A. Cordasco, "Anterior Cruciate Ligament Injuries in the Female Athlete," *Journal of Gender-Specific Medicine* 4(2001): 25–34.

CHAPTER 8: The Skin

1. K. Yano, L. F. Brown, and M. Detmar, "Control of Hair Growth and Follicle Size by VEGF-Mediated Angiogenesis," *Journal of Clinical Investigation* 107(2001):409–17.

2. D. A. Wrone et al., "Melanoma and Pregnancy: Eight Questions with Discussion," *Journal of Gender-Specific Medicine* 2 (1999):52–54.

3. The University of Michigan's Institute for Social Research conducts the Monitoring the Future survey, which is supported by the National Institute on Drug Abuse (NIDA), National Institutes of Health. For latest survey data, visit the NIDA website at http://www.drugabuse.gov.

CHAPTER 9: Pain

1. E. Libman, "Observations and Individuals' Sensitiveness to Pain (with Special Reference to Abdominal Disorders)," *Journal of the American Medical Association* 102(1934):335–41.

2. P. D. Wall and R. Melzac, eds., *Textbook of Pain,* 3d ed. (Edinburgh: Churchill Livingstone, 1994), 1–7.

3. R. B. Fillingim and W. Maixner, "Gender Differences in the Responses to Noxious Stimuli," *Pain Forum* 4(1995):209–21.

4. D. A. Marcus, "Gender Differences in Chronic Headache in a Treatment Seeking Population," *Journal of Gender-Specific Medicine* 3, no. 6 (2000):50–53.

5. National Institutes of Health, "Illness and Pain," *Gender and Pain* (April 1998).

6. Ibid.

7. Ibid.

8. Ibid.

CHAPTER 10: Sexual Dysfunction

1. H. A. Feldman et al., "Impotence and Its Medical and Psychosocial Correlates: Results of the Massachusetts Male Aging Study," *Journal of Urology* 151(1994):54–56.

2. E. Laumann et al., "Sexual Dysfunction in the United States: Prevalence,

Predictors and Outcomes," *Journal of the American Medical Association* 281(1999):537.

3. S. R. Leiblum, "Sexual Problems and Dysfunction: Epidemiology, Classification, and Risk Factors," *Journal of Gender-Specific Medicine* 2(1999):41–45.

4. E. Frank et al., "Frequency of Sexual Dysfunction in 'Normal' Couples," *New England Journal of Medicine* 299(1978):111–15.

5. S. G. Nathan, "The Epidemiology of DSM III Psychosexual Dysfunctions," *Journal of Sex and Marital Therapy* 12(1986):267–82.

6. P. J. Fagan et al., "Sexual Dysfunction and Dual Psychiatric Diagnoses," *Comprehensive Psychiatry* 29(1998):278–84.

7. R. J. Mathew et al., "Sexual Dysfunctions in Depression," *Archives of Sexual Behavior* 11(1982):323–29.

8. A. Kearney-Cooke and D. M. Ackard, "The Effects of Sexual Abuse on Body Image, Self Image and Sexual Activity of Women," *Journal of Gender-Specific Medicine* 3(2000):54.

9. S. R. Davis, "Androgens and Female Sexuality," *Journal of Gender-Specific Medicine* 3(2000):36.

CHAPTER 11: The Lungs

1. E. H. Baldini and G. M. Strauss, "Women and Lung Cancer: Waiting to Exhale," *Chest* 112(1997):229S–34S.

2. S. Basavaraj, "Smoking and Loss of Longevity in Canada," *Canadian Journal of Public Health* 84(1993):341–45.

3. D. R. Gold, X. Wang, et al., "Effects of Cigarette Smoking on Lung Function in Adolescent Boys and Girls," *New England Journal of Medicine* 335(1996):931–37. Centers for Disease Control and Prevention, "Tobacco Use Among High School Students—United States, 1997," *Morbidity and Mortality Weekly Report* 47(1998):229–33.

4. M. Pope, M. J. Ashley, et al., "The Carcinogenic and Toxic Effects of Tobacco Smoke: Are Women Particularly Susceptible?" *Journal of Gender-Specific Medicine* 2(1999):45–51. E. A. Zang and E. L. Wynder, "Differences in Lung Cancer Risk Between Men and Women: Examination of the Evidence," *Journal of the National Cancer Institute* 88(1996):183–92.

5. Action on Smoking and Health (ASH), *Statistics: Women and Tobacco* (October 27, 2000).

6. A. M. Jette, H. A. Feldman, and S. L. Tennstedt, "Tobacco Use: Modifiable Risk Factor for Dental Disease Among the Elderly," *American Journal of Public Health* 83(1993):1271–76.

7. S. C. Stewart, "Tobacco and Women: Trends and Strategies for Quitting," *The Doctor Will See You Now* (2000); online at http://www.thedoctorwillsee younow.com/articles/womens_health/smokingcess_4/.

8. J. Yoshida et al., "Secretion of hCB/[beta]-hCG by Squamous Cell Carcinoma of the Lung in a 31-Year-Old Female Smoker," *Japanese Journal of Clinical Oncology* 30(2000):163.

9. K. R. Chapman et al., "Gender Bias in the Diagnosis of COPD," *Chest* 199(2001):1691.

10. K. Tan et al., "Modulation of Airway Reactivity and Peak Flow Variability in Asthmatics Receiving the Oral Contraceptive Pill," *American Journal of Respiratory and Critical Care Medicine* 155(1997):1273.

11. L. Rees, "An Aetiological Study of Premenstrual Asthma," Journal of Psychosomatic Research 7(1963):191.

12. A. K. Singh, R. K. Cydulka, et al., "Sex Differences Among Adults Presenting to the Emergency Department with Acute Asthma," *Archives of Internal Medicine* 159(1999):1237–43.

13. Jerry Krishnan, "Race and Sex Differences in Consistency of Care with National Asthma Guidelines in Managed Care Organizations," *Archives of Internal Medicine,* 161(13) (2001): 1660–68.

14. L. H. Ferry, telephone poll, Foundation for Innovations in Nicotine Dependence, Loma Linda, California, October 2000.

15. B. Dautzenberg (Office Français de Prévention du Tabagisme), paper presented at the Eleventh World Conference on Tobacco or Health, Chicago, August 2000.

16. W. Lawrence Beeson et al., "Long-Term Concentrations of Ambient Air Pollutants and Incident Lung Cancer in California Adults: Results from the AHSMOG Study," *Environmental Health Perspectives* 106(1998):183.

Index